HOUSE CALLS

•Stories from Thirty Years of
Rural Medicine Among the
Amish and English•

Gary Yarbrough, M.D.

Dear Reader:

The following twenty-one stories are from actual house calls I have made in three different states during my thirty years of practice as a rural family physician. Some are humorous, some sad, some sublime. I have changed the names and in a few cases altered circumstances slightly to protect privacy as much as possible. I sincerely hope that with these measures - and with some of the details blurry enough in my memory - no one will recognize themselves or acquaintances, or take offense if they do.

It is a shame the house call has largely disappeared. In making a house call the doctor can see the patient in his or her "natural surroundings", and in seeing the home, come to understand much more about the daily life and stresses the patient experiences. Usually the patient will be more relaxed than in a clinic setting and tell the doctor things he or she would not mention in the office. Moreover, given the new highly technologic changes in medicine with electronic medical records, new coding systems, and ever more government and other third-party interference, making a house call helps to reorient the physician's focus on just the patient. I feel very strongly that having the opportunity to make house calls truly completes a physician's experience in the practice of medicine.

I hope you enjoy these stories as much as I appreciated having had the chance to live them.

Gary Yarbrough, M.D.
Parsons, Kansas
March 2013

Table of Contents

Bad Breath

Five-thirty A.M. A telephone call this early would likely be from an Amish patient, probably wanting me to give them an appointment for today - as if I kept the appointment book at home by the bedside. At times these early morning calls seemed annoying, but deep down there is that subtle form of pride that takes pleasure in feeling needed.

"Hello," I said sleepily, then heard in reply the voice of Jonathan. He had called last evening about Rebecca, his wife, who was having a fast pulse, ranging from 110 to 120, as best as Jonathan could count being unused to the exercise. This morning he reported that Rebecca still has a fast pulse but now her breathing is very fast. She can't seem to get her breath. He said this had begun about four o'clock this morning and seemed to be getting worse. He wanted me to come out and see her right away. I agreed.

Jonathan and Rebecca had moved to this new Amish settlement with their five children just a couple of years ago. Such a move is often very difficult for an Amish family. The Amish live separate from the "world". Their world is their extended family and community. The fact that her parents and brothers had also moved here eased somewhat the pain of leaving behind a lifetime of friendships to be part of this new community. It had not been an easy transition for Jonathan and Rebecca. Jonathan was now working much of the year in construction. His jam and jelly business was of course seasonal, but the bills were not. On top of that his berry garden had suffered terribly from the drought of last year, and they had spent much of their savings on the rural water bill. With the construction work Jonathan might have to travel three or four hours away to the construction site, but it was work, and he was good at it. Now they would have a doctor bill, too.

As I was dressing sleepily but quickly, I began pondering possible causes for her fast pulse and rapid breathing. Naturally the first categories to come to mind were heart and lung disorders. Could she have a abnormal fast heart rhythm? That would explain the fast pulse and perhaps the shortness of breath as well. It didn't seem likely to me, as I was putting on my shoes, since Jonathan had found a pulse rate far lower than what one would usually see in that case.

God forbid she had had a blood clot to the lung causing all this. She wasn't really overweight (though she thought so), and having come through five pregnancies and deliveries without such problems her having one now was not very likely, either. She didn't even have varicose veins in her legs, at least not superficially, I thought, as I reached for my coat and headed out to the car. The little PT Cruiser I drive is just right for making house calls, with plenty of room in the back for my black bag and the soft luggage I use to carry medications to dispense. There is even room for a minor surgery kit, too.

It was still quite dark as I drove away, and though the winter air was crisp, the roads were dry. There was no traffic out this early, so I could continue thinking about Rebecca's symptoms and what could be their cause. Jonathan had mentioned she had had no fever so infectious causes were unlikely, though still possible. As I had almost twenty miles to go to get to their house, I had plenty of time to create in my mind a good list of possible diagnoses. Yet about half way there I realized how silly I was being. Had I a medical student doing a rural rotation with me, I would gently inform the student that any mental list of diagnoses he or she made would be a nice intellectual exercise but rather premature - all we had to go on was rapid pulse and breathing, both of which could be caused by any number of things.

As I turned into their lane, I was relieved I had made it there without running into any deer. This pre-dawn light was just the thing for hitting a deer and ruining a perfectly good early morning, not to mention my car. Jonathan met me at the side door that opened into the old garage which he had converted into his jam and jelly factory. He would usually wait for me to come in and go up the steps into the main part of the house. Meeting me right there told me how worried he was about his wife.

Rebecca was sitting in the old recliner chair that Jonathan usually used. There she was able to lean back and get a deeper breath than if she was sitting bolt upright or lying down. It was obvious she was very short of breath, and I knew her well enough to see the fright in her eyes. I checked her pulse quickly; it was almost 140. She was not moving, conserving all her energy to breathe. She said she was very weak and felt dehydrated though she had had no vomiting or diarrhea. She had eaten a small amount last night; it made her feel worse.

Opening my bag, I dug out the blood pressure kit, placed it on her left arm, and began pumping up the pressure. It was then that I noticed her breath. She had an overpowering bad odor to her breath, pungent and sickly sweet. When I mentioned this, she acknowledged having noticed it too and was embarrassed about it. Now I knew what was causing her fast pulse and rapid breathing. As I finished taking her pressure, which was quite low, I asked if she was thirsty. She said that for the last week she felt like she couldn't get enough to drink no matter how much she tried. Then I told her, " You have been urinating huge amounts, too, haven't you?" "Yes," she replied, "but that was because I was drinking so much for my thirst."

The mystery was now clear. Her symptoms were not due to a primary heart or lung problem at all. They were in response to another serious problem, the new onset of diabetes mellitus with diabetic ketoacidosis, know as DKA. Normally, with adequate insulin, the body uses sugar as a preferred fuel, producing waste products of carbon dioxide and water. In the absence of insulin, fat and protein become the primary fuels for the body, producing waste products of acids and ketones. In ketoacidosis the sugar and ketones give an odor to the breath that you never forget once you have smelled it.

As weak as Rebecca was, with the powerful odor to her breath and her low blood pressure, I knew we had no time to waste, as untreated DKA is a fatal illness. I told Jonathan I was going to take her in my car to the hospital right away. He agreed and would make arrangements for family to watch the children; he would join her later at the hospital.

Jonathan helped me get Rebecca into my car. I was glad as I drove off that we had only a few miles of rural gravel road until we hit asphalt. The rest of the drive back to town and the hospital was all paved. Once I hit the pavement, I was able to drive as fast as I dared. Several days later Rebecca told me I had scared her with my driving that morning; she had never gone so fast in her life. I told her we were even then, for she had scared me, as sick as she was. On the way to the hospital I called the ER to let them know a bad case of diabetic ketoacidosis was on the way to them. Thus they were able to get prepared the things they would need for her initial fluid replacement and insulin infusion. Once she was safely in the ER bed, I was finally able to breathe a sigh of relief.

In DKA the elevated level of acid in the blood (acidosis), is the most accurate measure of the severity of this illness, not how high the blood sugar rises. The normal blood pH, the measure of acidosis, is 7.35 to 7.45. The lower the number, the more acid the blood. Anything below 7.00 is considered severe, and hers was 6.93. The lowest I had ever seen before - and the patient still survive - was 6.85. Now I was glad I had driven so fast!

It has been a few months now since Rebecca was in the hospital. She's home on insulin as well as a pill for her diabetes. Fortunately she took seriously our instructions on diet and exercise, and she has been able to lose weight and reduce her insulin requirement. I only wish that my other diabetic patients would do that well. Yesterday she called to tell me she was doing great but just had just one small question. She said, "With my last babies I did not see the obstetrician until I was seventeen or eighteen weeks along. How about now?" Sadly, I informed her that insulin dependent diabetes is one of the trickiest things to manage in pregnancy; she would have to see the obstetrician right away.

Patients like Rebecca keep it interesting, even after thirty years of practice!

The Jesus Sign

In the 1980s I had the privilege of meeting and working with a remarkable woman who called herself Rosie. A stout black woman in her sixties (she would never tell her real age), she had spent most of her adult life as a nurse, then midwife, serving the same rural black community in which she had grown up. Rose was her middle name. She did not use her first name as she was named after a spinster aunt whom she didn't like. Strange, how we can reject for perfectly logical reasons the decisions our parents made for us, yet feel hurt and confused when our children do the same to us (for clearly silly reasons)!

When I first moved to town and began my practice, Rosie came to me to ask if I would be willing to work with her. She was cordial but reserved at first, sure of herself but unsure of this new young doctor. Most of the doctors in that community who did obstetrics would have nothing to do with her. Perhaps this was because of malpractice concerns, perhaps racial prejudice, or perhaps for other reasons related to a history of which I was unaware. In any case, I realized right away that this woman had delivered far more babies than I had at that point in my career. I readily agreed to assist her with difficult home deliveries. I was able to do forceps deliveries, which she could not, and I felt she could teach me things not taught in residency. She did.

The first case for which she called me out to assist was an unmarried teenage girl laboring at home. She lived with her mother and younger siblings in a part of town most whites don't see. Rosie felt this baby might need a forceps delivery due to its size and the size of the mother's pelvis. I was willing to trust Rosie's experience. Unfortunately, as is the case with too many of these girls, the baby's father was not there. I greeted the mother at the door and entered to find out more from Rosie. It was at first difficult to hear her over the repeated shouts coming from the bedroom in the back of the house: "Oh God! Oh Lord! Oh Mama!" Our patient was repeating this litany as frequently as her contractions came, always in the same sequence without, I supposed, any particular theological significance to that order: "Oh God! Oh Lord! Oh Mama!"

Rosie informed me that this family was not poor enough to qualify for welfare assistance, and since the mother had delivered her babies at home, the daughter was going to do the same. However, unfortunately for us, the daughter did not inherit her mother's stamina and pain tolerance. We had a patient out of control. Rosie had already tried everything she knew from her years of experience to calm her without much success. Yet given Rosie's experience, I was surprised that she did not know exactly how far along our patient was in her labor. Rosie related how the girl would almost climb right up the headboard of the bed when Rosie would try to check her. "You can try to check her if you want, but I wouldn't advise it," she said. She led me into the bedroom and introduced me to our patient, a wide-eyed, obviously frightened, and untrusting young girl. I carefully explained to her precisely why and how I needed to check her, in as calm and reassuring a voice as I could, just as I had been taught in residency. She climbed right up the headboard for me, too, and I was also unable to check the progress of her labor. Rosie and I left the room together, both of us wondering how this girl had ever managed to get pregnant in the first place.

Sitting once again in the front room, sipping the coffee our patient's mother had fixed for us, I asked Rosie how we were ever going to know when our patient was ready to begin pushing. "Don't worry, Doc," she told me, "We'll know when we get the Jesus sign," her heavy-set body shaking with a silent chuckle. I thought about asking her what this sign was, as I had never heard of it, but not wanting to sound as inexperienced as I felt, I said nothing. She probably sensed my thoughts as she just nodded at me and said, "You'll see. It shouldn't be long now." As we drank our coffee, I knew that I had been taught the science of obstetrics, but I sensed that here was a master of the art of obstetrics. After a while the repeating trilogy of shouts from the bedroom seemed to fade to the background, much as one might stop attending to traffic sounds coming in an open window.

Suddenly I spilled my coffee as I heard a much louder, more piercing screech, "Oh God! Oh Lord! Oh Ma... JEESUS!!" "That", said Rosie calmly, "is the Jesus sign." We arose together and went into the bedroom. Clearly our patient was feeling the urge to push and was now willing to work with Rosie and push with her contractions. Though the baby's head was a bit large for the mother's pelvis, Rosie was able to deliver a healthy baby girl without my having to use forceps. Our patient had done surprisingly well with pushing in labor, given her initial complete lack of control.

I had little to do to assist in that delivery, but Rosie insisted I charge a house call fee for having come, and the patient's mother agreed and paid me. As I drove home, I couldn't help wondering if the new baby might grow up to be the next generation in this family to opt for home delivery. I also couldn't help feeling grateful that I had learned something new that they don't teach in university hospital training - the Jesus sign.

Blonde Hair

The only other time Rosie called me was for another teenage girl named Millie, who was having her first baby. Rosie knew the family well. This girl was a good student in high school, was very popular, had many friends, and was involved in a wide range of activities. In time it had become obvious that at least one of those activities went beyond the normal definition of extra-curricular!

Rosie had followed her throughout her prenatal care. She was impressed that Millie had done an outstanding job of taking care of herself during this first pregnancy, and Rosie was not one to be easily impressed. Millie had not used tobacco or alcohol, watched her weight and diet, and kept every one of her scheduled appointments. She had taken prenatal classes at a hospital in the nearby larger town and had read several books about prepared childbirth. After all this Millie was very intent on having a home delivery, and the decreased costs associated with that were a bonus. Her thorough preparation, the absence of any prenatal problems, and the presence of a very supportive family made Rosie feel Millie would be an ideal home birth candidate.

Millie had handled early labor with ease. She had tolerated her contractions well, relaxing and resting well between them. The first stage of labor is when regular uterine contractions bring about thinning and dilation of the opening of the womb. Once dilation is complete, the mother can then begin pushing with each contraction to bring the baby down the birth canal.

This young girl was ready. She knew what was happening. She understood labor and managed to do a great job of pushing initially. Then as Rosie continued coaching her through pushes, Millie seemed to lose control. She had advanced the baby's head part way down the birth canal but then stopped. As the pressure of the baby's head became greater with each contraction, she just stopped pushing with them. That's when Rosie called me.

I met Rosie at the front door of the family's home. Rosie quickly filled me in as she led me to the room where the delivery was to take place and introduced me to the patient. Shortly after I entered the room the next contraction began. Instead of pushing with it, all Millie could do was pant, turn her head from side to side, and say, "I can't, I can't, I can't..." There are some things you just can't learn from reading a book, and this was one of them for her. Rosie and I both tried our best to help her calm down and work with her labor, but our efforts proved futile. Millie would just thrash her head about with each successive contraction, insisting she "couldn't".

Donning a sterile glove, I checked Millie through a contraction and found the baby's head would descend a little in the birth canal, only to go back with uterine relaxation. Clearly she needed help at this point. Rosie and I were agreed that the use of forceps would help get Millie to the point of delivery. Rosie poured sterile saline over the forceps to moisten them, and I inserted them as I had been trained to do. With Millie's next contraction I was able to bring the baby's head down to where she could be delivered the rest of the way by Rosie. However, now with the increased pressure of the baby's head, Millie was even more actively asserting, "I can't, I can't..." I then said in my most reassuring tone, " Sure you can! The baby's ready to be born. I can see the top of its head. Why, it has a full head of blonde hair!" I worked hard to keep a straight face and not laugh. Rosie stared up at me in surprise.

I had gotten their attention. Millie stopped saying, "I can't", drew herself up onto her elbows, looked me hard in the eye, and said, " What? You jivin' me!" After a short moment of silence I replied, "Now that you're listening to me, there's only one way for you to find out. With your next contraction push right through all that pain and pressure, and we'll have this baby delivered." The next contraction came, she pushed with it like a champ, and out her baby came.

Millie was immediately up on her elbows again, straining to see her newborn son. I admit I did hold him a little low while suctioning his mouth and nose as Rosie clamped off his cord. I finally held him up for Millie to see her beautiful baby boy with his full head of black hair. She let out a deep sigh and laid back down on the bed for the last part of labor, the passing of the placenta. That was uneventful.

Several weeks later I met Millie, and she told me that at first she was a little mad at me for having tricked her. She said she later realized I had actually helped her through what was, for her, the toughest part of the birth of her son. I told her I was truly pleased to have been able to help her, and we parted friends. head of blonde hair? worried? Yet I've always wondered - a full What was the reason she was so

Coma

Most of us use the word "hysterical" to refer to something imminently humorous. Medically, however, the term was used to describe symptoms involving the nervous system in which major bodily dysfunction is caused by psychological stress. Many have heard of someone with such overwhelming stress that they are suddenly paralyzed or blind. These people are by no means "faking" their symptoms. They truly are suffering these conditions, but the cause is mental not physical. The full term for this used to be hysterical conversion reaction, as the psychological stress is "converted" into physical symptoms. Now it is called by another less descriptive term. I think the older name fits it better. I had never fully realized how dramatic these reactions could be - and how desperately these people really needed their symptoms - until a house call one holiday morning.

As can often be the case, I was the only doctor available in our small town that morning. I was called by a very upset lady to come to her house to see her son. They were unable to wake him from his nap. She told me he was breathing normally and had a good pulse, but he did not respond to talking or even shaking to awaken him. Though I was not his regular doctor, I told her I'd be there shortly. Sometimes in a small town one can't be too particular - neither them nor me.

When I arrived at the house, I was ushered into the living room. There I saw a man appearing to be in his mid-thirties and apparently asleep on the couch. I, too, could not get him to respond to talk, touch, or even what should be mildly painful pinching. There was no response at all. The family informed me that he had had no history of diabetes, head injury, seizures, or other neurologic symptoms in the past. He had apparently seemed completely normal before lying down for his nap.

I proceeded to examine him in detail, carefully looking for neurologic clues that might distinguish a true coma from an hysterical one. There are several tests in a physical examination that will give widely different results for these two conditions. His exam quickly made it clear that we were dealing with a conversion reaction. Since he seemed in no immediate danger, I then turned to the family for more information about him.

The family told me he had been a hard-drinking, wild-living truck driver. His first wife, fed up after five years of drunkenness and irresponsibility, divorced him and took custody of their children. After that he had gone on a terrible binge, losing first his driving job, then one job after another. After finally "hitting bottom" he began attending AA meetings, rebuilt his life, and now was working again as a trucker, this time a teetotaler. He had even met a young woman with whom he had fallen in love. He had invited her to meet him at his parents' house for the holiday dinner, at which time he was going to announce their engagement.

It sounded like all was well with him at last; however, his ex-wife had found out about his new ways and wanted very much to try to get back together with him. She had always remained close with her in-laws for the children's sake. When his mother found out he was coming home for the holiday, she invited the ex-wife and children to come over for dinner, too. When he arrived at the house, he told his parents about the guest he had invited and that he had a surprise for them. His mother then told him about whom she had invited to come to dinner. At that point he said he was tired and went into the living room to lie down on the couch. By the time all the guests arrived, he was found in the comatose state.

Given all this information, now I had to decide what to do for this man. The local hospital would not accept him for admission as there was no psychiatrist on staff to treat mental disorders like his. Rural psychiatric resources were rather scant. I placed a call to the on-call mental health worker and waited for a call back. The state hospital, though far away, was one option, but it was the very last place most state residents would ever want to go. I decided to use this to my advantage.

Sitting by him on the couch, I loudly informed the family that this was an hysterical coma, a conversion reaction due to the stress he felt at the two women being there at the same time. I "reassured" everyone that these conditions do not often last very long. If he did not "awaken" in fifteen minutes, I would have to arrange his transfer by ambulance to the state mental hospital since no closer hospital was equipped to deal with psychiatric problems like this. After making this "authoritative" announcement I rose from the couch and watched my patient from across the room.

Exactly fifteen minutes later he "woke up" and slowly sat up on the couch. I carefully explained what had happened to him, wrote him a prescription for a mild tranquilizer, advised him to contact his own physician after the holiday, and left him in the company of his "extended" family. Everyone seemed relieved he was back with them again. The on-call mental health worker did finally call back and concurred with this management strategy.

Driving home I felt pretty pleased with myself for what I thought was an elegant solution to a difficult problem. I thought the family had seemed impressed with this young doctor who had so quickly pulled their loved one out of a coma. Such vain thoughts did not last long, however. That evening his father called to tell me his son had been taken to the local hospital with a self-inflicted gunshot wound to the head. I was stunned. Later I found out he had been transferred to a neurosurgical center where he died the following day.

Apparently this man could not handle the conflicting emotions of his new fiancé, his ex-wife, and his children all coming together over a holiday dinner. His conversion reaction coma gave him a way out of having to deal with that stress. When I took that away from him, he found final refuge in suicide. I'll never forget that house call, where I learned how crucial their symptoms can be to those suffering from conversion reactions.

Emma

John Erly and his two brothers all served in the Civil War. Thanks to the grace of God and some bad enemy marksmanship, all three survived. After the war none of them had much, but they pooled their resources to begin a wholesale-retail furniture business to help rebuild the South. In ten years they were wealthy men. John married that year, and for a wedding present had a beautiful two-story brick home built for his bride out in the country near town. He felt that a city was not a "fitting" place to raise children. His second present to his bride was that she could select whatever she wanted from the store or warehouse to furnish their new home, and in that fine home their four children were born and raised, the youngest being Emma, born in 1880, when Rutherford B. Hayes was our president.

Emma saw all her older siblings marry and leave before she married a young man herself. They had planned to live in the big family home until her husband had earned enough to build their own house, but that never happened. The very year they were wed he left to serve with the Rough Riders in the Spanish American War and was killed in Cuba. It wasn't long afterward that Emma found she was pregnant. Her son was born in the same house where she herself had been delivered. After the loss of her husband and the birth of her son, Emma had talked with her parents about attending the Normal School, a two-year teacher's college, and they agreed she should. Once she graduated, she returned to begin teaching in the local rural school, a career that spanned over forty years and that she dearly loved.

When Emma was seventy-five years old, a power company was buying up land for a major transmission line to be built in the near future. That power line would run right through her home. By then Emma was retired, hypertensive, and had had a slight stroke. She had suffered the loss of her husband, all of her immediate family, her career, and now partial use of her left arm. She was not about to suffer fools gladly and lose her family home, too. As she had taught most of the residents in the county, she had a lot of support throughout the community for resisting the power company. Realizing the fix they were in and with local resentment growing, they offered Emma what they thought was a great compromise. The power company would buy her home and property, but they would allow her to continue to live there until she died. Emma accepted. Little did they know how long they would have to wait.

I was first called to the house to attend Emma when she was one-hundred two years old. It had been twenty-seven years since she had signed the contract with the power company, and they were still waiting! When I received the call from her housekeeper, she asked me to come to the back door of the house. At first I wondered why I was told not to use the front door. That afternoon as I drove into her lane, I immediately saw the reason. The front porch was in terrible disrepair and not safe to use. Since the back door was in good condition, Emma had not thought it necessary to spend the money to fix the front since, as she put it, "It belongs to the power company anyway."

I met her housekeeper, Mrs. Johnson, at the back door which opened into the old summer kitchen, itself not in the best condition. However, as I entered the main part of the house, my jaw dropped. Here were magnificent antiques looking brand new. Even the wallpapers showed little aging. I was walking through rooms so well kept that it looked like I had stepped back in time to the Victorian era, except for the presence of electric power, which had obviously been a later addition. I noticed also that there were no old gaslight fixtures; piped natural gas had not been available in that rural area in 1875 when the house was built. Mrs. Johnson led me up the polished oak staircase to Emma's bedroom. She was lying propped up with several pillows on an old-fashioned feather bed. Against the wall opposite the foot of her bed was an original, like-new Edison phonograph. Above it was a cabinet full of the wax cylinders to play on it; it still worked. Emma greeted me pleasantly, extending her hand, the thin skin almost translucent. I saw right away that her age clearly exceeded her weight. As I began my exam in detail, I found that her blood pressure was not well controlled, her urine output was decreasing, and her deer-thin lower legs and ankles were swollen with fluid.

When I finished, it was clear she needed major changes in her medication. Her kidney function was compromised not only by age but by her old medication regimen. Having written her new prescriptions
and drawn blood for testing, I was ready to leave, but Emma insisted we first have a cup of tea and visit. It was during those visits that I learned the history you have just read. After forty-minutes I left, much more knowledgeable about Emma and her past and promising to return in a week to recheck her.

When I returned the following week, the swelling in her ankles had resolved, and her blood pressure was much better. She reported that her "kidneys had recovered", and she did indeed look much better. This time she was sitting up in a chair. Emma was bent forward from osteoporosis, the thinning of the bones and loss of height that occurs with advancing age, and it looked worse with her sitting up. She was in good spirits, though, and reported having had no trouble with side effects from the medicines I prescribed. Her blood tests had shown poor kidney function, so I drew another set to see just how much recovery had actually occurred.

Two tests are most commonly used to evaluate the kidney. The BUN, blood urea nitrogen, will vary from hour to hour. The normal range is around 10-20. Hers had been 50. The creatinine is a longer term test, varying week to week. Its normal range is 0.8-1.6. Hers was 3.5. Her second blood test showed a BUN down to 30 and a creatinine down to 2.5. These numbers were better, but her kidney function was nonetheless permanently impaired due to her advanced age.

Over the next two years I made several calls on Emma. She always insisted on the tea, and while we sipped it, she would tell me more stories about her past. I looked forward very much to my visits with her just to hear those stories. She had lived through so much American history - the Spanish-American War, World War I, the world-wide 1917 influenza pandemic, the Great Depression, World War II, and much more. She had seen transportation go from horse and buggy to the space shuttle, and she had seen two presidents assassinated - McKinley and Kennedy. Yet in all that she told me, she said the saddest day of her life was the day she walked from the church to the cemetery in the funeral of her son, who had died of "old age" at eighty, when she was ninety-eight.

I think Emma must have finally decided she had had enough; it was her turn to go. She called to thank me for all I had done for her and to let me know she would not be needing me again. At the time I thought she had just decided to see a different physician. It wasn't until later that I learned she simply stopped taking her medications. Within a month she had had a massive stroke and was gone at the age of one-hundred four.

It seemed like the whole county turned out for her funeral, including me. She is still the oldest patient I have ever attended.

Breath Sounds

There was an ice storm that afternoon followed by a light but constant snowfall. Dianne, my wife and office nurse, and I drove home together. It took twice the usual time along the twisting river road and up the steep lane to our house. We had supper with our four children and were settling down for the evening when the phone rang. It was Flora calling for her husband, Beau. Many folks in that rural eastern Kentucky county thought of Beau as a hard man. I did not. He wasn't mean but tough as nails and yet gentle. It was an interesting combination of personality traits born of a poor rural upbringing and World War II.

Beau was born on a hard-scrabble farm in one of the county hollers rarely disturbed by outsiders. While eighteen year-old Beau was helping his father cut tobacco, Hitler was invading Poland. Beau enlisted in the Army and served in Europe throughout the war, returning afterward to be stationed in Louisville while awaiting his discharge. Though he had never shrunk from a fight growing up, Beau had seen too much fighting and killing in the service. It changed him, as it did so many soldiers, and he had come home with a different understanding of fighting and peace.

While in Louisville Beau checked up on his savings. Beau had had his eye on a piece of bottom land hidden deep in the hills near his home that the owner had promised to sell him when he got back from the war. No one back then said "if", just "when". He had spent almost nothing during his years in the Army and now had enough to buy the land, build a home, and resume his life. That was what Beau had planned. What he had not planned was meeting Flora, the

27

woman who would be by his side for the rest of his life. Flora was from a wealthy family, folks who would ordinarily not associate with those from deep in the eastern hills. The two met at church, fell in love, and eloped, taking the train back to his beloved hills to begin their life there. I'm not sure if she ever communicated with her family again after that.

Beau was a hard working man, and in a few months had built a three-room log home, a barn, a chicken coop, and had plowed the flat part of his land and planted his first tobacco crop. Tobacco brought the most money per acre, especially important where flat acreage is at a premium. Beau and Flora worked the farm together, raising several children as well as the tobacco. They had been working their farm for over twenty years when we moved to that area to begin my first medical practice after residency. Flora met us at church that July; later that first year she invited us to their farm for Thanksgiving dinner. That was our first invitation to someone's home for dinner since moving there, and we eagerly accepted.

Thanksgiving morning we drove down the winding river road to the sign pointing to their dirt lane, then followed a mile-long winding path along the creek running out between the wooded green hills until we came to the farm, up a rise from the creek. We met Beau, Flora, and their other guests at the cabin home as our four children went off to play with their two youngest children still living at home. My wife was amazed at the dinner Flora had prepared, as it was all cooked on an old wood stove, yet all came out done at the same time: a ham, a turkey, five pies (two of them fruit), homemade candied yams, homemade cranberry sauce, mashed potatoes with turkey gravy, hand-made stuffing, split-pea soup with ham, bread and dinner rolls all ready for the table simultaneously.

We had a great dinner, but it was there that I initially noticed Beau had a bad cough, more than the usual smoker's cough; twice he had to leave the table with coughing spells. The following month he went to the VA hospital where he was diagnosed with an aggressive lung cancer and began treatment with chemotherapy and radiation. His doctors knew this was only palliative, not curative, but I'm not sure Beau understood that. He came home having lost a lot of weight and quite weak from the treatment. Being home and eating Flora's cooking helped him regain some of his strength, but not many weeks after coming home he developed a fever. That's when we were called to come see Beau that icy night.

The six miles along the icy river road were tense, but Dianne and I managed to reach their lane without sliding off the road. The dirt lane had some ice but wasn't as slick as the pavement, though the falling snow and that already covering the lane made it difficult to follow. I was grateful that we had been there before so I knew where we were going. Unfortunately, we didn't quite make it to the house. As the lane rose from the creek to the house, it turned slightly to the left. Twice we slid backwards down to the creek. One of the boys got their tractor and pulled us the rest of the way up by the house. As we got out and walked carefully toward the front door, we had to pass by the chicken coop. Dianne sank above her ankle in snow, mud, and chicken poop. She later laughed about it and told me she had been surprised at how warm it felt, but at the time it wasn't very funny.

Flora met us at the door and led us to the main room of the cabin where Beau was lying very still on the old couch, his face ashen and damp as if misted with sweat. Dianne quickly rechecked his temperature while I found out more about how Beau had been doing. His temperature was 102.5°. He had become progressively short of breath the last few days but did not have a fever until that morning. Beau wouldn't let her call me until that evening, when he was finally too weak to argue. Now he was too sick even to sit up to be examined.

On examination I found his throat was dry and slightly reddened, and his neck veins prominent. However, by far the most worrisome finding was his breath sounds heard with the stethoscope. Two different abnormal sounds could be heard. The first was loud rattling in the right lower lobe area; these sounds are not uncommon in pneumonia. He also had tubular breath sounds, similar to the sound of breathing through a snorkel or other long tube. These sounds indicated that there was at least one fairly large airway being pinched off. Given Beau's history, this pinching was likely due to cancer.

Having worked in the VA hospital during my recent residency, I knew the number for the main VA switchboard and quickly dialed it. When the operator answered, I identified myself and asked for the oncology resident on call, the specialty that deals with cancer. After a short time the resident answered, and I related to him what was going on with Beau. I told him I thought Beau had pneumonia behind a recurrent cancer and needed to be sent to the VA hospital for admission. Tired from his already long day, and perhaps a bit annoyed at having to workup another admission, he asked with a tinge of sarcasm, "What does his x-ray show? What's his blood count?" As measured as I could, I replied, "Friend, I am standing on the hard dirt floor of this man's log cabin. Even if I had x-ray and lab machines, there is no electricity here to plug them in." There was a rather long pause before he answered, much more softly, "Sorry. Send him to us."

I called the county ambulance, a ten-year old Cadillac vehicle that the funeral home maintained. They came but made it only as far as we did; they also were towed up to the house by the tractor. I helped the crew get Beau onto the ambulance cart and provided them with the written note I had prepared for the on- call resident. Dianne and I visited for a while with Flora before we drove home, relieved to get back safely and that we had been able to get Beau to the care he needed.

The following week I was surprised to receive a telephone call from that same resident with whom I had spoken that night. He told me that Beau's chest x-ray and CT scan had confirmed my diagnosis of pneumonia behind recurrent cancer. He complimented me on having diagnosed this with just Beau's history and a stethoscope. Beau, he said, was receiving antibiotics and more treatment for the cancer, but so far had not responded well.

Beau died at the VA hospital. We had lost a friend.

Spinal Meningitis

This was the third time in as many months that Mrs. Jackson had called the office insisting that I come "right away" to see her four-year old son, Peter, whom everyone knew as Petie, her first and only child. She resisted bringing him to the office since he was usually "too sick", and she worried about his sitting in the waiting room among "all them other sick people". On each of the previous two times I had come to see him at the home, just a few blocks from the office, I had found a child suffering from no more than a cold, without even a trace of fever. When I had given her this diagnosis, she accepted it begrudgingly. She seemed unsure if I knew what I was doing, as if I had missed something gravely serious in her son's evaluation. Both times she told me she would call again "as soon as he was worse". I supposed he had not gotten worse, as both times she had not made those second calls. Later I found out that instead she had taken him to the older doctor in town, who had prescribed an antibiotic for what was clearly a mild cold. Interestingly, she would not call him initially as he would flatly refuse to make a house call to see her son.

Now this morning she had called again, asking me to see him once more. She told my nurse that he was sicker than he had been all year. She dared not bring him to the office "with all those germs. In his rundown condition who knows what might happen." The nurse related all this to me. I held out for an office call. Mrs. Jackson declined as Petie was "too sick" to leave the house, and would I come to see him there soon. Though I felt she really didn't trust my medical judgment and would likely see the older doctor again when she wasn't satisfied, I finally agreed to see Petie during the lunch hour. I didn't want to take the chance that he might really be sick this time, and being the new doctor in town, I could use the money. Mrs. Jackson did pay her bills.

At lunchtime I drove over to the Jackson house. It wasn't the finest house in town but was by no means the poorest. The family was doing well financially even though Mrs. Jackson had quit work when Petie was just one year old and had never returned. I was told by others that she had informed her employer she must stay home with her son full time as he simply couldn't be put in day care.

I felt rather sorry for young Petie. He was rarely allowed to play outside and even less often have other children over to play. This didn't seem to bother Petie. He was a happy child, content to play alone much of the time, yet always pleased to see someone visit their home. When I arrived, he recognized me right away and ran to the dining room to sit on the chair where I had examined him before. I set down my bag on the dining table, took out the tools I would need to check him, and began to examine him. Having seen me twice before and not having been hurt, he didn't mind. His mother stood right beside him.

I checked his temperature - no fever, then his ears, throat, chest, and belly, all of which were normal. His nose, though, had a little clear fluid coming from it. If this went backward instead of forward, it would tickle his throat and start him coughing. That was all. Once again, it was painfully clear that I had been called to see a child with no significant illness. Now what to do about it.

Twice before I had explained to Mrs. Jackson that Petie was not significantly ill, and twice she had apparently rejected my reassurance that he would be fine. Finally it dawned on me to try to find out why she was calling a doctor to see her son for so little. This time I thought I'd better use a different approach. I said nothing while I was putting my things back in my black bag. Finally, packed and ready to go, I said, "Mrs. Jackson, Petie has a runny nose. He may be getting a cold or just have allergies. But he certainly has no illness serious enough to justify your calling me to check him and then have to pay for a house call. It isn't good for either of us. Why are you calling me like this?"

"You don't understand, Doctor," she said pleadingly. "When he was jes' a year old we'd almost lost him. He acted jes' like this, and it was the spiny mighty Jesus!"

It took me a moment looking at her with a blank stare to figure out what she had just told me. Petie had had "spinal meningitis". This was what made her so sensitized to his least symptom. This was also, in a way, my own fault. I had failed to obtain a thorough enough history to find this out the first time. I then sat down with her for a long talk about how a runny nose or a slight cough could amount to nothing more serious, and that such mild symptoms could indicate any number of things, perhaps the least likely of which would be meningitis. She seemed to understand.

Maybe I didn't do any better job of explaining things this third time. Perhaps she still didn't trust my judgment, and I could understand that, since I had failed to get a full history

34

on Petie. For whatever reason, she no longer called the office requesting house calls. But at least I had learned two things - never omit taking a thorough history, and a new term - "spiny mighty Jesus."

First Swiss

Most people, when they hear the word Amish, think of the Pennsylvania Dutch riding down a rural road in an enclosed buggy. Yet the Amish are as diverse as any other faith group with many different sects, and within each there are communities whose Ordnung, or community rule of living, varies widely. Among the most traditional and restrictive are the Swiss Amish, who came from Switzerland and bordering areas where the Swiss dialect was spoken. They drive open buggies with no protection from the weather, no "message phones", propane, air-driven tools, or any power machinery in farming. Everything is still done with "horsepower".

The Swiss Amish first settled in the eastern part of Indiana, mostly notably in Adams County near the towns of Geneva and Berne. To this day they speak a dialect unique in this country to their communities, though I was told people still speak it in Switzerland. Interestingly, the Swiss Amish say they can understand the Pennsylvania Dutch, but the Dutch can't understand them; yet the Pennsylvania Dutch speakers say the same about the Swiss! From Indiana the Swiss expanded to Missouri, then seven years ago they began a new community just twenty miles from here. I had served several Amish communities in Michigan and had read extensively about their customs and way of life. My wife and I had formed many good friendships with the Amish patients there. We both looked forward to meeting the Swiss Amish and providing them with medical care.

The first Swiss I was called to see was an elderly gentleman having trouble breathing. Noah was a deacon, one of the elders of the church, a position not of elevated status but rather of service and responsibility; such duties are a real burden to bear. He had a Santa Claus beard (minus the mustache) and hair cut in the Amish style with long Ben Franklin hair in the back. Noah knew quite a lot about hospitals, doctors, and medicine, much more than the average Amish man. As a young man he had been drafted. For religious reasons of conscience Amish are given alternative service when drafted, and Noah was sent to work in a hospital in Indianapolis. Most of his time there he was assigned to work in the mental ward, and he had many stories and jokes to tell about that experience. He picked up a great deal of knowledge about medical care in general during those years and afterward returned to his community.

Noah had lived in this area just nine months when I was first called to see him. He had a history of adult-onset diabetes, high blood pressure, and coronary disease. He was already taking multiple medications for these problems including nitroglycerin for the chest pain, but now he was running through a bottle of nitroglycerin quite rapidly. He had had a coronary stent placed five years prior. At that time he was told there were several more blockages, but they did not require stenting then. Now he was experiencing progressively worsening chest pains with activity and shortness of breath. His breathing was getting so bad that he could lie down to sleep only a couple of hours before he awoke with shortness of breath and had to sit up; he then would try to sleep in his chair. He initially denied having swelling in his legs, but on examination it was obvious he had that, too. His heart sounds told me he was in bad heart failure, his lungs were wet with fluid, and he was in serious trouble with angina and heart failure. He, of course, knew it but would minimize it to others.

Taking his medical history, I learned that he had had joint replacements in addition to the cardiac stent, all of which were very expensive As he put it, "I've cost the community too much already." It was clear that he needed more coronary stents. The lesser blockages noted five years ago were now critical themselves. Yet Noah would not agree to go to the hospital for this.

This was the first of many times in working with Swiss Amish that I would face the same ethical dilemma. The standard of care in medicine was to stabilize him at our local hospital then transfer him to Joplin where cardiologists could provide the definitive care he needed. However, Noah would not accept that. I decided I would try to help him within the parameters he would allow.

Noah told me he had "Medicaid payback" in Missouri for his previous coronary stent. This allowed him to be charged at Medicaid rates. The community then paid back the state and canceled the Medicaid. I told him I would see if this could be done in Kansas and also check with the cardiologists in Missouri about what they could offer. I drew blood for lab testing; it was not easy. Noah reassured me, telling me it had always been hard to get blood from him. I wrote new prescriptions for him, hoping the adjustments in medication would help. I promised to return the next day.

The next day he said he was feeling better. The blood tests showed his diabetes had been well controlled; those medications need not be changed at this point. His cholesterol was elevated; he would resume medication for that, medication which he had stopped on his own. There was one test, though, that was not good at all, the heart failure test. The normal for this test is under 100; his result was over 2,500, indicating the most severe level of heart failure.

I told Noah I had found out that Kansas has no "Medicaid payback" program like Missouri. I also told him that I had arranged for him to go to Joplin for the stents he now needed. The hospital and cardiologists had agreed to do this at Medicaid rates for him. However, he still refused. I nodded, remarking, "That's what I thought you would say." He looked surprised and asked, "Then why did you bother to arrange all that?" I answered, "I figured you would still refuse, but there have been a few times before when I've been wrong." He chuckled and thanked me for my efforts on his behalf, even though he was not willing to do it. As he felt better and his lungs sounded better, I made arrangements for him to see me at the office in a week. He could use the local hospital patient van if necessary. I gave him the telephone number for that.

A week later he was clearly not better. A chest x-ray showed significant congestive heart failure, and an EKG showed a recent heart attack. Still Noah was not willing to go to the hospital. Again I adjusted his medications and gave him an intravenous injection to make his body dump more fluid. I planned to see him again at home in three days. He didn't make it that long. His shortness of breath and chest pain worsened; two nights later, he consented to come to the local hospital. He was admitted and given vigorous treatment for the heart failure. He responded very well and went home after three days, able to walk without gasping for air or needing nitroglycerin. We had made progress.

Noah always had a good sense of humor and a twinkle in his eye. He appreciated being able to go once again to "work frolics" (barn raisings) even though he could only supervise and visit. This was very important to him. As someone once put it, visiting is the Amish national sport. With time, though, the coronary blockages and his diabetes progressively worsened. I had to start him on a long acting insulin, and for his shortness of breath he now required home oxygen. The usual way to do this is with an oxygen concentrator, a machine that pulls oxygen from the air for the level of inhaled oxygen the patient needs. However, that would require electricity, not available in his home. Oxygen tanks wouldn't last long enough for regular use. We decided to go with liquid oxygen, which one of our local medical oxygen suppliers kept on hand. By using this occasionally during the day as well as during the night, he could go one or two weeks on a thermos of liquid oxygen.

Eventually, even with all this, we were unable to keep Noah going. He finally became so short of breath that once again he was brought to our local hospital for care. This time, though, he was transferred to the Joplin hospital where he underwent a cardiac catheterization. This showed such extensive disease that bypass surgery was his only option. He declined it, as I suspected he would. He died the next day, content that he would not cost his community any more. In his culture death from this world to begin life in the next was easier for him to accept than being a burden to others.

Burns

Joseph and his wife Elizabeth had moved to the new Swiss Amish settlement the year before with their children, all nineteen of them. They had had twenty, but one died many years prior. Of course, they could use neither electricity nor propane to heat the water needed for washing dishes and laundry, and for bathing that many people. So Joseph had come up with his own unique system for heating enough water for the entire household.

Joseph had purchased a huge cauldron, similar to those you've seen in cartoons or old movies in which cannibals roast missionaries. His was big enough to hold at least four! The cauldron rested on a polygonal metal skirting with a door for putting in the wood, vent holes for the fire, and a side hole for the stove pipe that vented out high on the wash house wall. A swing arm attached to a supporting beam of the wash house was fitted with a chain fall to the cauldron. This mechanism permitted the cauldron to be raised and swung easily to the side for cleaning out the ashes. A fire begun in late afternoon would give the whole family enough hot water to last all evening and into the next morning. This seemed to be the perfect system for providing adequate hot water, until that fateful blistering July afternoon.

That day their daughter Mattie was sent to the wash house to light the fire. Mattie was a lovely eleven- year-old girl who eagerly helped with the household chores. She had done this particular chore many times. Using a sprayer bottle, she would wet each piece of wood with kerosene before placing it under the cauldron. Once enough pieces had been put in, she would light it with a match and close the fire door. Within a few hours hot water would be ready to carry inside for washing the dishes.

This particular day, however, her brothers had found a yellow jackets' nest in the field they cultivated that morning. After lunch they took the kerosene sprayer with them to burn out the nest. When Mattie went out to start the fire, it was gone. So, to get her chore done, she put several pieces of wood under the cauldron, picked up the can of kerosene, and began to splash it over the wood. Unfortunately, there were still live embers there from the previous day's fire. The kerosene erupted in a flash explosion.

Hearing the explosion, everyone in the vicinity ran to the wash house. There they found Mattie, badly burned and her blue polyester dress on fire. Her mother, Elizabeth, quickly put out the burning dress and removed it. Her father carried her into the house, ran to a neighbor, and called me. I advised him to cover her with cool wet cloths, and we would come right away. My nurse quickly canceled the remaining appointments for the day. At that time I had a medical student doing a rural rotation with me. She helped gather together the supplies we would need. We loaded up my PT Cruiser, and the three of us left for Joseph's farm fourteen miles away, each of us worried about what we were going to find.

When we arrived, we carried our supplies into the main house. There on the long dining table Mattie was lying with the cool cloths on her. She was in considerable pain. Her siblings were crowding around the table waiting to see what we were going to do. The first thing, with the help of their parents, was to shoo them all outdoors. I had some pain tablets in my medication bag and dosed Mattie with this right away. I then began an examination to identify where she was burned and how extensively.

Her eyebrows were gone and her face as brown as a Mexican. Her eyelids, however, were not burned; you could see pale white wrinkle lines where she had winced. Her face, left shoulder, armpit, arm, and forearm were all blistered as was the front of her chest. There were blisters like giant worms on the tops of all her fingers. She had more blisters scattered on both legs from the buttocks to the toes, some areas missing the uppermost skin layers. Some areas had traces of melted blue polyester incorporated into the blisters. Fortunately she had no third-degree burns of the full thickness of the skin.

All three of us then worked on Mattie for almost an hour, cleaning all her burns with sterile saline, removing as much of the polyester as we could, then dressing each of the burns with Silvadene burn cream and sterile dressings. When we were done, we took careful note of how many supplies we had used. We would need to order much more over the coming weeks. I gave Joseph her prescriptions for pain medication and an antibiotic to help prevent infection. Elizabeth and he were instructed to keep Mattie drinking enough water that her urine was as pale as lemonade and to keep her cool but not shivering. Joseph placed her bed under the shaded front porch window where she would have a slight breeze. We helped him get her into bed and promised to return the next afternoon at 3:00 PM. I asked her mother to give her a pain pill an hour before we would come.

The next day we brought a small cooler with us filled with popsicles. The medical student handed them out to the siblings on the front lawn and asked them to stay outside to eat them. This gave Mattie the privacy she needed. Mattie said that she had good pain relief from the pain pills, but she was not looking forward to having her dressings changed. We helped her hobble to the dining table where we examined her again. Her face and lips were now swollen so that she could barely open her left eye. As gently as we could, we removed all her dressings. There were large areas of loose dead epidermis, the top layer of the skin, over many of the burned areas. Fortunately, there was no pus or foul odor to any of the wounds. Those on the lower buttocks and upper thighs were redder that the others, but there was still no sign of a full-thickness burn. We trimmed off as much of the dead skin as possible, cleansed the wounds with sterile saline, and reapplied sterile Silvadene dressings to all the burns. We always saved a popsicle for Mattie to have when we were done.

For the next two weeks we drove to the farm each afternoon to attend to Mattie. Each day there were more cards and notes taped around her window sash from her school friends. Each day the burns were healing a little more, and Mattie was able to walk better. She had remained without fever until the evening of the fifth day when it spiked up to 102°. She had no throat, chest, or urinary symptoms, and her wounds that day still had no bad odor or bad drainage coming from them. I called in a prescription for a second antibiotic. After the second dose her fever came down and did not return.

After two weeks all of the blisters were resolved, and there was no more dead tissue needing to be trimmed away. At that point Mattie's mother felt that she would be able to do the dressings. She had watched carefully how we did it and felt she could do the same. The next day we supervised while Elizabeth removed the old dressings, cleansed the burns, and reapplied new dressings; she did an excellent job. Joseph asked about B&W, or "burn and wound" cream, an Amish-made product highly touted for healing burns. He wanted to try it. I suggested they could, but let Mattie decide which seemed to do better. Mattie preferred the Silvadene.

It took several weeks for all of Mattie's burns to heal completely, and we continued to see her weekly. Throughout that entire time Mattie never once complained or fought us as we treated those burns, though she would cry when something hurt. It has now been almost four years since that terrible July day. Looking at Mattie now, one would never know she had been so badly burned. She does have some minor scarring at the left elbow, but it does not restrict her use of the elbow and doesn't bother her. To this day I regard Mattie as the bravest patient I have ever treated.

Values

Amanda was just two days old. She was born at home in near record July heat, the youngest of Peter and Leah's sixteen children. Her delivery by the midwife had been uneventful, and no one else in the family was sick. Yet on her second day of life Amanda was not doing well. She had become fussy and would not nurse as well as she had initially. Her father went to the store and bought her special newborn formula, but she would not take that either. I was then called to see the baby. I had a medical student on rural rotation with me, so my nurse, the student, and I drove out to their farm twenty-two miles from town. It was midafternoon on a 102° steamy July day.

We arrived at the farmhouse and went inside to see the baby. It was stiflingly hot in the front room where it seemed very dark after coming in from the sunlight. Peter had a thermometer on the wall inside; it registered 98°. Leah was sitting in a chair with the new baby on her lap. Most of the other children were standing about in the room to see what we were going to do. Our first task was to take the baby's temperature. It was 104.2° rectally. I examined the baby and found pneumonia in the base of the right lung with wheezing. This child was in extreme danger. We gave Amanda a dose of acetaminophen and convinced Peter and Leah to bring the baby and come with us to the office for further care. They agreed, and once we had Amanda in Dianne's air conditioned van, her temperature began falling.

By the time we got back to the office Amanda's temperature was down to 101°. We obtained a chest x-ray, which confirmed the pneumonia, and a culture to try to identify what bacteria might be the cause. The next problem was the question of hospitalization. In routine practice Amanda would be admitted to a neonatal intensive care unit (NICU) and put on IV fluids and antibiotic. She would then gradually be switched to taking nutrition and fluids orally as she improved. The nearest NICU was in Joplin, about sixty miles away, and she would be sent there by ambulance or helicopter.

Unlike secular American culture, for the Swiss Amish this life is but a stepping stone to the next. This is not our true home, and we are to be careful stewards of what God has given us. Therefore, if a newborn is stricken with such a severe illness, there is a decision to be made about using all their resources for this one child or preserving them for everyone else. Often deciding on the former could impoverish an entire community given the high costs of modern medicine. "The Lord giveth , and the Lord taketh away" was understood; the death of a baby like Amanda might be in God's plan. Such a child would be soon back in heaven in the Father's arms. Moreover, the Swiss Amish were open to all the children with which God would bless them. Families of fifteen or twenty children were not uncommon. In secular American culture, by contrast, children are often seen not so much as a blessing as a burden. Abortion and artificial contraception are used to severely limit their numbers. Then the loss of a single child becomes a huge catastrophe.

Having worked with the Swiss for a few years, I understood their cultural values. Nonetheless, the choice not to send this baby to the hospital could be considered child abuse, ironically by those very same professionals who insist we must be "culturally sensitive" to those from other cultures. Somehow such people don't include a culture based on living out the Christian faith Biblically and simply. If I did not send Amanda to the NICU, there could be legal problems for us all.

I talked to Peter and Leah about how sick Amanda was and about the issues both ethical and legal regarding her care. They had lost a newborn in the past, and they did not choose neonatal intensive care then; they would not do so now. Both of them understood the possible consequences should Amanda not recover with home treatment, and both of them agreed to accept those consequences should Amanda die. The medical student working with me was wide-eyed at this discussion. She had never before met people whose culture allowed them to accept death simply as a part of this life, a mere doorway to heaven.

We prepared an antibiotic suspension for Amanda, gave her the first dose, and gave Leah the new dropper to use with it. We also provided them with a hand-held battery powered nebulizer and the medication for it. This enabled Leah to give Amanda breathing treatments at home even though there was no electricity. As we drove them back to their house, I talked with Peter about additional steps to take in caring for Amanda. They had the special newborn formula if Amanda would not nurse, and they had the medication for fever. I was worried about the house being so extremely hot in this July weather. Peter informed me that the basement remained at 80° during the day and cooled to 78° overnight. I suggested to them that Leah and Amanda live in the basement for the next week or so, and both parents agreed. When we arrived back at the house, Leah went directly to the basement with Amanda while Peter and the older boys carried a bed and table downstairs to the basement for them. As we returned to town, the van was quiet as we were each lost in thought.

The next day we drove back to the farm early in the morning. Amanda was now eating much better, even nursing again. Her fever was down, and she was breathing much better. She still had lung congestion but no wheezing, as the nebulizer had helped her. The culture had grown out staphylococcal bacteria, and the next day we learned it was sensitive to the antibiotic I had prescribed, "sensitive" meaning it would kill the bacteria causing Amanda's pneumonia.

After another three days Peter called me from an English neighbor's phone to let us know that Amanda no longer needed the nebulizer, but now she had a white rash in her mouth. Once again we drove out to the farm. Amanda had thrush as I had suspected. This time I could show the medical student how to calculate the dose of the antifungal medication, which for Amanda came to almost 300 mg for the usual 14-day course. Instead of calling or writing a prescription for the commercial liquid preparation, at a cost of over sixty dollars, I showed her how to use a mortar and pestle to grind two 150 mg tablets into a fine powder. This was then mixed with fruit juice to make 30 ml of suspension. Amanda would take 4 ml the first day, then 2 ml each day thereafter for the fourteen-day treatment. This reduced their cost to eight dollars for the two generic tablets. The suspension we prepared resolved Amanda's thrush nicely.

I think the medical student learned many things that summer about the delivery of health care and about dealing with values markedly different from those she would encounter in the university hospital setting. At least she went home understanding a Christian culture she had never before experienced, and how medical care could be delivered in the home at a dramatically lower cost.

Shunt

David and Maggie were not among the first group of Swiss Amish to move here. Others had been here over a year before they came. David's father was a very stern, controlling man, and David had many of the same traits. I suspected that his father played a role in David's delay in moving, as well as his decision finally to do so. His younger brother, Moses, had talked with David about the idea. Moses and his family had moved here a month earlier, so there was at least some family here when David arrived.

Besides having to cope with his father's ways, life had not been easy for David and Maggie. Mary, the second of their fifteen children, had been born with a neural tube defect in her spine, the spinal canal being left open. This can range from the harmless "spina bifida occulta", in which there are no symptoms or neurologic defects, to the "myelomeningocele" in which the spinal cord, spinal nerves, and the surrounding membranes (meninges) are protruding out on the back under a thin layer of skin. In these severe cases there is a flaccid paralysis of the body below the defect with no reflexes or sensation; they cannot feel touch or pain. Often the urinary bladder and bowels are affected, and many of these children have club feet and other defects. Finally, most of these children have a blockage of the normal flow of cerebrospinal fluid through the brain and down the spine. They develop hydrocephalus, commonly called "water on the brain", which produces increased pressure, leading to brain damage if not relieved.

Mary had a lumbar myelomeningocele at birth. She had undergone multiple back surgeries as an infant. These operations repaired the back defect, but her neurologic problems were permanent. She was paralyzed below the level of the myelomeningocele, leaving her unable to walk or urinate normally. Her parents were taught how to use catheters to empty her bladder. She had a club foot for which she also had surgery. Later as a toddler she developed a deep infection in that foot and ankle. Due to her lack of sensation this progressed to infection in the bone, and her foot had to be amputated. Finally, Mary had a shunt placed as an infant, a thin tube with one-way flow that relieved the pressure on the brain, draining the spinal fluid into the abdominal cavity.

When Mary was in her early teens, she began having severe headaches. The doctors at the university hospital found her shunt was not working. She then had another surgery to replace the shunt. Amish children are usually very shy and soft-spoken around the "English", and also being an anxious teenage girl facing this surgery, she did not speak much; her parents did most of the talking for her. Unfortunately, as a result, it was recorded in her medical record that she was mentally retarded.

Like most Swiss moving to a new farm, they lived initially in the "machine shed". This was a large one-story barn-like building in which the family would live until the main house was built. Later it would be used for storing the horse-drawn farm machinery, thus the name. Filled with sixteen people and all their household goods, the shed was crowded.

The preceding autumn before their move Mary had bad headaches. Her doctors found her shunt was fine, but she had a urinary tract infection. Antibiotic for that infection cured her headaches, too. Now she was having headaches again. Her mother was concerned that she might have another bladder infection. I was called to see Mary for these headaches just a month after they had moved into the machine shed.

Mary was now twenty-four years old. She spent most of her day in a wheelchair. She had an artificial left foot but did not use it much since she was unable to walk. It was more cosmetic than useful. Her headaches had returned, but this time she also felt pains in both shoulders, numbness in her face and hands, blurry vision, and decreased hearing. Mary had no fever, but her blood pressure was elevated, which could be due to increased pressure on the brain. She was able to answer all my questions with clear, intelligent speech; she was obviously not mentally retarded. When I told her this, she smiled from ear to ear and nodded in agreement!

Mary's urine showed signs of infection. A urine culture confirmed this, and she was begun on an antibiotic that would be effective against the bacteria causing that infection. Due to the presence this time of the other symptoms besides headache, I made arrangements for Mary to have a shunt study done at our local hospital. These shunts have a small reservoir bulb under the scalp. A tiny amount of radioactive tracer was injected into the reservoir. A nuclear scan showed radioactivity in the abdomen within an hour; the shunt therefore seemed to be working.

Over the next several days Mary seemed to improve. Her headaches were less intense, but the numbness in her face and hands, the pains in her shoulders, and the blurry vision did not go away. After a week her urine, which had been clearing, now was cloudy and had a bad odor. This time the urine culture showed a bacteria resistant to multiple antibiotics. In addition, Mary was now having trouble holding her head up, and at times she choked with swallowing.

Mary's worsening neurologic symptoms proved her shunt was not working, even though the nuclear study a week ago showed it was. It was time to get her to the neurosurgeon. This was what her parents had feared. They were already financially stretched in getting established on a new farm, and now they would be facing huge medical expenses. Sadly, there was no choice. I had already done all I could with home care. They agreed to the referral to neurosurgery.

I called the neurosurgical group in Joplin, as they were the closest. They did not want to take her case when they found out she had no insurance. I discussed the situation with David, Maggie, and Mary herself. We all agreed to try to get her to the university hospital in Columbia, Missouri, where she had all her previous surgeries. The neurosurgical resident on call there asked why I wasn't sending Mary to a closer facility. When I related to him the response I had received, he agreed to accept her case.

Now the problem was how to get her there. An ambulance ride of over 300 miles was out of the question. Fortunately, there was a Catholic couple who had heard of my work with the Amish and had volunteered to help if needed. They owned a full-sized conversion van which would be big enough for the task at hand. If ever there were a case where their help was needed, this was it. I called them and filled them in on what was happening. They agreed immediately to take Mary to Columbia, a five-hour drive one-way. They even refused any payment from David for the ride. Instead, David would make the husband a bent hickory rocking chair; that chair is now a prized possession in their home.

Mary's shunt was indeed not working, and she had it replaced. After the surgery her neurologic symptoms immediately began subsiding. Within six weeks the numbness, headaches, neck weakness, and pains were gone. She has remained well since then. To help her parents pay for her medical expenses, Mary assembled a cookbook of favorite Amish recipes interspersed with stories and bits of wisdom. Pretty good work for a "mentally retarded" girl! The cookbook has sold well.

The Youngest

It was a pleasant June Sunday evening when I got the call to see Emily, a 16 month-old Amish girl. Her father, Herman, told me she had been well until that weekend when she began running a fever, coughing, and wheezing at times. I had seen her twice before, at seven months of age and again when she was one year old, both times for ear infections. It seemed likely that she might have this again, but with the cough and wheezing there was likely more going on. I told Herman that we would be out shortly. Dianne, my wife and my RN, said she would come along with me. We went to the office to pick up Emily's chart, my doctor bag, and the dispensing medications. Since Herman had mentioned wheezing, I decided to bring along one of our two battery-powered nebulizers as well. We then drove the twenty-two miles to his parents' farm, where Herman had told me the family was visiting.

We drove into the lane to find the grandparents, parents, and Emily sitting in the evening shade of a large oak near the side door of the grandparents' home. Emily ran to Mattie, her mother, at our approach. Of course, like any child that age, she did not want to be examined by the doctor. However, with Mattie's assistance, we got the job accomplished. It helped that I had seen her twice before and not caused her any discomfort so she was wary but not crying.

Though she had had a fever according to Herman, it was only 98.1° under the arm by the time we arrived. Emily had a red right eardrum, but the left was normal. Without the noise of crying it was easy to hear the wheezing in her chest and fortunately, the absence of the sounds of pneumonia. This time she had an asthmatic bronchitis and another ear infection. We mixed the liquid antibiotic for the infection and began her on nebulizer treatments with a bronchodilator medication. I suspected she might be infected with Haemophilus influenza, a bacteria that can cause both problems. Dianne explained to her mother how to dose both medications. After that we visited for about a half hour. It was growing dark, so we said goodbye, drove back to the office to drop off the chart and supplies, and then drove home.

Two days later Herman called to report that Emily seemed to be doing much better. The nebulizer treatments has quieted her breathing, and her fever was gone. She was eating better as well. I advised Herman to have her complete the course of antibiotic, and that I could come by at a later date to pick up the nebulizer when they felt she no longer needed it. That seemed to me to be the end of this episode of illness for Emily. I was wrong.

Herman called four days later to report she had "taken a turn for the worse" in the last day and a half. Though the nebulizer had initially helped her, it was no longer working, according to him. Now she was breathing even harder than before she began the medications, and the breathing treatments made no difference. In addition, she wouldn't eat well though she readily drank liquids. I advised Herman that it seemed clear that now something else was happening. Perhaps she had been infected with another organism not sensitive to the antibiotic and had developed a pneumonia or other complication. Whatever it was that was causing Emily so much trouble, it was obvious that another house call was not what she needed. I advised Herman to take her to the emergency department of our local hospital.

The doctor on duty examined her and ordered a chest x-ray and blood tests. To everyone's surprise the blood tests showed that she had a blood sugar over four hundred! She was in diabetic ketoacidosis, digesting fat and protein instead of glucose as her body had stopped producing insulin. This causes the accumulation of excess lactic acid in the blood. Her hard breathing, called Kussmaul respirations, was her body's effort to correct the acidosis in her blood by exhaling as much carbon dioxide as possible, since lowering the carbon dioxide level reduces its acidity. This type of diabetes - type I - is thought to be from an autoimmune mechanism in which the immune system makes antibodies against the pancreatic cells that make insulin, destroying them and eliminating the body's insulin production. Why this happens we do not yet know.

The pediatrician on call was asked to see Emily. He began the process of stopping the ketoacidosis by giving her IV fluids and insulin. He then arranged for her transfer to the children's hospital in Kansas City, where she was cared for by pediatric diabetologists (specialists in diabetes) and begun on a regimen of home insulin shots based on finger-stick blood sugars. Her parents were educated extensively about this disease and given telephone numbers they could call at any time for help in managing her care at home. I had thought my job in examining her was tricky. Now her parents had to do her fingerstick glucose testing and insulin shots three times a day.

Emily is now an active two year-old and seems to have accepted the blood tests and insulin shots. At least she will accept this from her parents! The pediatrician who had seen her in the emergency department later told me that in all his years of practice, Emily was the youngest patient with type I diabetes he had ever seen.

Kinky Hair

I had read that when Amish patients find a doctor they trust who practices medicine in a way that respects their values, they will come from long distances to see that physician. Yet I was still surprised to find I was seeing patients from Missouri and Pennsylvania while practicing here in southeast Kansas. One of the most remarkable cases I have seen, though, came from just across the border in Oklahoma. The husband, Eli Borntrager, called me initially asking if I would make a house call to see his wife. When I asked him what was going on with her, he told me she was having problems getting pregnant. He related that they had been married "a while" but had no children. She was not having regular periods. I told him that I would be happy to see her, but that I could not make a house call to treat her as I was not licensed to practice medicine in Oklahoma. I suggested she come to the office at least for the first visit, and I would see what I could do.

Two weeks later I heard from him again. This time Eli wanted to know if I would see his wife at the home of an Amish family they knew here in Kansas. I informed Eli that I would be able to do that since it does not matter so much where the patient lives as where I am licensed to practice. I also let him know that house calls are not usually scheduled but done after regular hours or on an emergency basis any time. He seemed pleased that I would see her if they came up to Kansas, but he was not sure how they might set this up with their friends here. Eli then told me as long as he had to hire a driver to bring his wife to Kansas, he might as well bring her to the office. We set up an appointment to which she came with her husband and both of her parents.

Priscilla Borntrager was a pleasant twenty-seven year-old Amish lady who had been married to Eli for several years without having any children. She had never been pregnant as far as she knew. Her periods didn't start until rather late at age sixteen, and they had never been regular. She frequently would skip months at a time. Six months ago she was seen in Oklahoma for abdominal pain and had removal of a small ovarian cyst and what turned out to be a normal appendix. She did not know if the doctors had seen any other abnormalities with her reproductive system through the laparoscope. She told me that as far as she knew, none of the other women in her family had this problem. In addition she told me she had always been a "slow thinker" but had managed to finish school, completing eighth grade, the usual Amish level of formal education. Perhaps it was for this reason rather than shyness that her mother was giving me most of Priscilla's history. When I asked Priscilla if I could assist her with anything else, she asked if I could help with her hair; it would break off and never grew longer than a few inches. For an Amish woman her hair "is her glory" as St. Paul says in the Bible. They never cut their hair short. Thus this short hair was a constant source of embarrassment for Priscilla. Finally, she reported having occasional "hot flashes", but she never had any type of dryness problems with marital relations or other menopausal symptoms. She did occasionally get headaches with reading, but she attributed this to her "old glasses".

I began her exam with the scalp and hair. Her hair was brittle, the longest strands only four inches. Her scalp appeared normal. Her skin was somewhat pale, but her mother said she had always looked that way, and Priscilla nodded in agreement. Her ears, nose, and throat were all normal. Examination of her neck revealed no thyroid mass or overall enlargement. Her chest exam was normal with no wheezing or sounds of congestion. Her heart exam revealed a regular rhythm with no murmurs or other abnormal sounds. Her abdominal exam showed the scars from the laparoscopy with no other significant findings - no mass, tenderness, or organ enlargement. As Priscilla had had a pelvic exam and ultrasound just six months ago when she had the abdominal pain, I asked if Priscilla could sign a release to get the records from those examinations rather than repeat them. She was quite eager not to have that exam again and agreed. Finally, I notice that Priscilla had what is called "spoon nails". The fingernails are concave and look like a spoon from the side. Her mother said she had had finger nails like that since birth. Priscilla said her toenails looked the same way. Neither she nor her mother were aware of anyone else in the extended family with nails like this.

After the exam I told Priscilla and Eli that I was not sure what was causing her problems. I told them I thought we needed to start with a hair sample and some basic blood tests, and they agreed. Priscilla allowed me to collect a few hairs for examination. I then drew blood for thyroid hormone (T4), thyroid stimulating hormone (TSH), a blood count, serum estrogen level, and follicle stimulating hormone (FSH), a pituitary hormone of the reproductive cycle. These tests would tell me about her pituitary, ovaries, and thyroid, and if she was anemic. The FSH would be a start toward evaluating her reproductive system. I knew that an infertility clinic would do much more testing, and the specialists there would consider this a most inadequate workup. Yet the tests they would order are often quite expensive, and I was trying to diagnose her in the most cost-effective way and not run Eli into debt if I could help it. I did not set up another appointment for Priscilla but rather suggested I get back with them when the tests results were available, and I had had a chance to review her records from six months ago. They agreed.

After they left, I took one of the hairs she had permitted me to collect and looked at it under the microscope. What I found was very surprising. Her hair shaft had periodic kinks in it. It was at these points that the hair would break off. When her records came from Oklahoma, where she had had the laparoscopy, I found that the ultrasound report showed the small right ovarian cyst without any other abnormal findings. Her pelvic examination was likewise unremarkable except for right-sided pain. She had a normal appearing uterus, fallopian tubes, and ovaries other than the cyst. Her thyroid tests also came back normal, and her CBC was unremarkable with no anemia. However, her FSH was very high - in the menopausal range! Her estrogen was barely in the normal range. This suggested to me that Priscilla's pituitary gland was trying to drive the ovary as it should, but the ovary was not really responding. Why would this girl be menopausal at only twenty-seven years old?

Reviewing my dermatology text, I found that there were several different types of abnormal kinky hair. All were genetic and seemed to run in families. Yet Priscilla and her mother knew of no other relatives with this. I called the dermatologists to whom I normally sent patients. They wanted to see her hair, so I sent them a few strands in the mail. They called me a few days later and agreed this was a kinky hair disease of some kind. I decided to search the internet to find more information on kinky hair.

Typing in "kinky hair" in the search box gave me hundreds of web sites, most of them neither medical nor related to Priscilla's problem. I tried "early menopause" and "kinky hair" with the same result. After trying many such searches without success, I finally typed "Amish" and "kinky hair" in the search engine. This at last was it - several web sites for "Amish kinky hair disease". All of them referred to an initial research study done decades ago on an extended Amish family group in northern Indiana. Several individuals in the family had the genetic trait causing kinky hair. Also, the affected individuals had few if any children; most of them were completely infertile. Finally, the affected individuals were all described as "slow in school", attributed to a mild mental retardation associated with this genetic disease. This was our answer, and I couldn't wait to tell Eli and Priscilla.

The next day was Saturday. Dianne and I drove to their address; no one was home. On a hunch we tried her parents address, and found them there. They all stopped and stared for a moment, surprised we had come since I had said I could not practice in Oklahoma. I told them I was there to teach, not "practice medicine", so could we talk about what I had found. We went over her results and the printed materials I had brought. They were relieved to learn why Priscilla had been "slow" in school. Her father remarked that Priscilla's teacher would feel bad to learn she hadn't really been a lazy student but couldn't help it. While it was disappointing to hear she would most likely never have children, they were content to know finally the reason.

I was deeply gratified to have solved this mystery without spending hundreds or thousands of dollars investigating the cause of Priscilla's infertility. The kinky hair had been the key.

Hemorrhage

It was fortunate we were not busy in the office that hot July afternoon when the call came. It was the midwife for the Swiss Amish community asking if I could come out to see Lovina. She had just delivered her baby boy, but the placenta would not come, and Lovina was bleeding more than the midwife thought was right. I knew this seventy-eight year-old midwife, who had delivered more babies than all of the doctors in this town put together, certainly knew how to deliver a placenta. This was not a good sign. I assured her we would be right out to the farm.

I had met Lovina before in seeing her first child, now one year old, for a fever and ear infection. She was a quiet woman and soft-spoken, so much so that at times I would have to ask her to repeat what she had said. She had married Samuel two years before, a very outgoing young man; it seemed their personalities complemented one another well. Their house was one of the closer ones to town, so it took us only about ten minutes to arrive.

I met the midwife in the main room, and she escorted me to the bedroom where Lovina had given birth. She was lying very still, and though the July heat was oppressive, she was chilling slightly. What really caught my eye was how pale she looked, her skin like translucent marble. This was evidence that she had already lost way too much blood. I put on a pair of sterile gloves and pulled back the sheet to check her.

I was alarmed to see how much Lovina was still bleeding. I could see the flaccid umbilical cord coming out, and

67

around it a steady flow of fresh blood. I began to massage the uterus through the abdominal wall and then made one gentle effort to remove the placenta. It would not budge. It was immediately clear that this placenta would not be delivered here. It was even more obvious that Lovina was in serious trouble. As I was walking out of Lovina's room, I called on the cell phone for emergency transportation to the hospital.

I had seen Lovina's condition only once before. It had been almost twenty years, but I still remembered that Sunday morning delivery as clear as yesterday. That patient had had a normal prenatal course and a routine delivery. However, I was unable to get the placenta to budge. Instead she began to hemorrhage, losing even more blood than Lovina.

At that time I was in partnership with an older physician who also did surgery. I called him and insisted that he come at once. He was obviously irritated with me, asking where I had trained that I couldn't deliver a placenta, but he agreed to come. When he arrived, he too was alarmed at how much blood the patient was losing. By then her blood pressure was beginning to drop in spite of having her IV running in as fast as possible. He also tried to remove the placenta, and she began to bleed even more. At that point he ordered units of blood I had already set up to be given, and he had her moved to the operating room where he performed an emergency hysterectomy to save her life. I was praying that would not be the outcome for Lovina, knowing how much having many children meant to her and to Samuel.

While waiting for the ambulance to arrive for Lovina, I was able to contact the obstetrician in town to alert him about who was coming his way and what was happening with her. After I explained to him her condition, he agreed to see her right away. He would notify the emergency department to make sure he was called the moment she arrived. He asked if I could start an IV to help support her blood pressure, but unfortunately, I did not have that with me. I told him I would have the ambulance crew start one as soon as they came and run it wide open all the way to the hospital. Again it was fortunate that Samuel's house was so close to town; some of the Amish farms were over twenty miles away.

Once Lovina arrived at the hospital the obstetrician saw her right away and had her prepared for an emergency D&C to curette or scrape out the placenta. If this failed to work, hysterectomy would be the next option. Lovina also would receive several units of blood to restore her circulating blood volume. The IV fluid given by the ambulance crew had stabilized her blood pressure somewhat, but she was dangerously anemic from the hemorrhaging. Fortunately the D&C was effective in removing the adherent placental tissue and stopping her bleeding.

What Lovina was suffering from, as had my patient twenty years earlier, is called placenta accreta. The normal placenta will form interlocking "fingers" with the inner wall of the uterus with a thin layer of tissue between. This allows the baby to receive oxygen and nutrition from the mother. The normal placenta will separate spontaneously along that thin tissue layer after birth of the baby. This process of separation is aided by uterine contractions.

In placenta accreta the intervening tissue layer is absent, and the placenta can grow right into the muscular wall of the uterus. It will then not separate after the baby is born, and it even impedes the contractions of the uterus. How much the woman hemorrhages is due to several different factors - where in the uterus the placenta is attached; how deeply into the muscular wall it has grown; how much of the placenta is abnormally attached; and how vigorous the attempts to remove it manually. The condition occurred in one out of 7,000 deliveries before 1970 but now it is more common, up to one in 2500 deliveries. Fortunately, though, the incidence of maternal death from this is going down.

Lovina did not have to have a hysterectomy. The obstetrician was able to remove the placenta with the curette and preserve her ability to have more children. Unfortunately, though, she suffered from placenta accreta with the next two pregnancies. However, for those babies Samuel and Lovina had chosen hospital delivery. As everyone was aware of her history, the problem was immediately recognized and treated promptly, again with preservation of her uterus and the ability to bear more children.

Her next baby was born without complication, hemorrhage, or placenta accreta. God alone knows why.

Silo Falling

Sometimes people have asked me to come out for a house call when, with a little thought, they might realize how useless that would be. Indeed, sometimes the situation can be so desperate that a call to 911 for an ambulance ride to the hospital would be a better alternative. I must admit that there have been times I have been fooled in this regard, as the person calling me has minimized the severity of the situation or perhaps did not realize that it could be fatal. At other times I have been asked to come to the house when the person calling should know that I can't provide the care his or her family member needs.

One example of the latter occurred just a year ago. It seems Emanuel and his sons were building their silo. For those not familiar with farming, a silo is a tall cylindrical structure in which silage, or food for the farm animals, can be stored for feeding them through the winter. The Swiss Amish would find an English farm where the silo had not been used for years. Some of these had been neglected for so long that they actually had good-sized trees growing out the top! These old silos were made of slightly curved, interlocking concrete blocks, much like a child's toy blocks, but on a much larger scale. The pieces were held tightly together by heavy wires bolted around the circumference. The Amish would offer to take down the silo and haul it away at no charge to the owner. They would then take the pieces home and reassemble them to make a silo that would actually be used again. Any pieces left over could be used as stepping stones in the garden or to make a "sidewalk" from the house to the barn.

Emanuel told me his seventeen year-old son, Jacob, had been high up the wall of the silo on a ladder. He was bolting the wires tightly together and needed some more nuts and bolts. Emanuel had tossed them up to Jacob, but not closely enough to him. When Jacob leaned out trying to catch them, he fell off the ladder and landed on his arm. Emanuel asked if I would come out and check Jacob's arm. He felt Jacob might need an x-ray. When I asked why he felt that way, Emanuel said the arm was looking crooked, not at all straight like it should be.

As kindly as I could, I explained to Emanuel that a crooked arm definitely needed to be x-rayed and most likely was indeed broken. However, it just wasn't possible for me to fit an x-ray machine into the back of my PT Cruiser and drive it out to their farm. Moreover, even if I could somehow magically do that, there was no electricity on their Amish farm with which to operate it! I suggested he take Jacob to the hospital where it could be x-rayed, the broken bones set, and the arm put in a cast. Emanuel took Jacob to the hospital. The arm was indeed broken. The orthopedist on call came to see Jacob, reduced the fracture, and put him in a cast for six weeks.

Two weeks later I was passing by their farm after having made a call to one of their neighbors. I decided to stop and see how Jacob was doing. Emanuel was pleased to see me and admitted he had felt a little foolish after he had called me that day. He knew I really wouldn't be able to provide Jacob with the care he needed after that fall, but with the excitement of the moment he hadn't been thinking clearly.

Jacob's arm was of course still in the cast, yet he was already eager to get it off so he could do his regular chores again. We talked for a while about the healing process for a broken bone and how the normal time it takes for good healing is six to eight weeks in an adult. In some cases where the bones are thin with osteoporosis from aging, it might take even longer. Jacob was relieved that didn't apply to him.

Emanuel then told me about another silo building incident that had occurred when he himself was a young man. This silo was being built on a farm located on the main highway leading into the town. It was a warm spring when they began working on it. There was a slight rise between the base of the silo and the road, so the bottom of the silo could not be seen from the highway. Most people did not know it was being put up until the first rows of blocks had been assembled. Once it was high enough to be seen from the road, the project began drawing a crowd.

Each day as they worked the silo grew higher, and it seemed there were more "English" stopping along the edge of the road to watch them work. After they had the first thirty feet or so assembled, the crowd watching was getting so large, those doing the work felt a little uneasy about being stared all day. Finally one of them got an idea for some fun.

Going home that night, two of them asked their sisters to help them put together a scarecrow-like dummy, dressed just like one of them in work clothes, complete with a straw hat sewn onto the head. With several of them working on it together, the dummy was done in just a few hours. The next day they took it with them to work, keeping it hidden on the inside of the silo near the top where they were working.

By lunchtime there was a good crowd of "English" watching by the road. Emanuel, being one of the smaller workers, was about the same size as the dummy. He hid behind the rise at the base of the silo and signaled to those at the top. They suddenly dumped the dummy over the top and began yelling as loud as they could, like someone falling from a high roof. When the dummy hit the ground, Emanuel would get up onto the rise, brush himself off, and begin climbing the outside ladder back to the top.

Still, after so many years, Emanuel laughed himself almost to tears, remembering the shocked expressions on the faces of the "English".

Looking Amish

Although Dianne and I are faithful Catholics, you might think I was Amish if you saw me walking down the street. The haircut, beard, and plain clothing all would give you that impression. My brother-in-law, Michal, who practices acupuncture and Chinese herbal medicine on the west coast, was among those who could not understand why I chose to look this way. I explained to him that it was a huge advantage in treating Amish children. It's scary enough for any small child to have to go to the doctor. It doesn't help if the doctor looks strange to them, and it's even scarier if they can't understand a word the doctor says. Amish children do not become fluent in English until they have been in school a few years. Since I had learned enough dialect to talk with them in words they could understand and my appearance was not so odd to them, the children would not be frightened, and I could do a better exam on a child without fear.

In addition to that, I have found that people in the secular culture were actually more polite when one looks Amish. Moreover, someone wearing plain clothes sends a signal to others that this is a person who takes seriously their Christian beliefs and can be trusted. Since the basis of every doctor-patient relationship is trust, this is an extra blessing in the medical setting. Patients feel more comfortable and secure in confiding information than when I wore "English" clothes.

Even having explained all of this to him, Michal really didn't see the advantage until one autumn day two years ago when he was visiting here in Kansas. That morning I received a call from Magdalena, one of my Swiss Amish patients, whose little girl, Sarah, had burned her hands on the wood stove five days before. She had blisters on the palms and the fingers which her mother had been treating with B&W (burn and wound) salve that she had ordered in the past through the Budget, the national weekly Amish newspaper. At first, she said, the burns seemed to be healing well, but yesterday two of her daughter's fingers were turning red and looked infected. She asked if I could come out. I told her I would be out around noon and invited Michal to come along.

Having lived most of his life in cities, Michal appreciated the opportunity to drive out through the country to my patient's farm. He was surprised to learn that the Swiss have no indoor plumbing. The "heezlee", or outhouse, suffices. There is a water pump in the kitchen and a drain from the sink, but that is all. He said that was like going back to pioneer days. I told him that many of my elderly "English" patients remembered living just like that when they were small children, but they could not believe that there were people still living that way today. There are.

As we drove up the lane to the farmhouse, we saw Magdalena and her daughter coming out onto the front porch. As soon as she saw the car stop, little Sarah ran back into the house. I greeted Magdalena and introduced her to Michal. The three of us then went inside to the front room, but Sarah was nowhere to be seen. Her mother left us standing there while she went through the house looking for her. I asked Michal if he would look at her injuries and tell me how he would treat them with the Chinese herbs.

76

Before he could answer, Magdalena returned and sat down facing us with Sarah in her lap, looking fearful and clinging to her mother. I motioned to Michal. He said, "Good morning," and took a step forward. He stopped as he saw the little girl's eyes widen, grabbing even tighter to her mother. Michal stepped back and turned to me. I slowly walked up to mother and child, then squatted down and waited a bit while Sarah had her face buried in her mother's dress. As she slowly turned to look at me, I whispered to her, "Sarah! Vas ish latts?" ("What is wrong?") She looked me in the eye a moment, then silently held both her hands out to me, palms up, to show me where she had been burned. I could see all the blisters, several of which were decompressed and flattened. Two of her fingers were reddened and slightly swollen; they looked like they might be infected. I stood up smiling at Sarah, and she smiled back. I had seen what I needed to see with neither tears nor struggle. I dispensed a sulfa antibiotic for Sarah to be sure to cover her for a staphylococcal infection, and we left.

As we started back to town Michal shook his head, still amazed at what he had seen. He told me he would never have believed it had he not seen it. "Now," he said, "I understand why you look and dress as you do. When she held her hands out for you to see them, I about fell over! I was wondering how hard it was going to be to check burned hands in such a young child, and I've never seen the like."

I explained to Michal that this was not the way such visits would go when I first began treating the Swiss Amish. However, as I came to look more and more Amish, and particularly as I learned their dialect, it gradually became easier to interact with and examine the little children. Now it was uncommon to have a child be frightened of me. Besides, I told Michal, Amish dropfall trousers are much more comfortable - no belt squeezing you around the middle. Just ask any farmer wearing overalls!

Paralysis

Christian Yoder was really sick. His wife, Amanda, called to tell me that he had had diarrhea and vague abdominal pain for over a week. He had felt weak for several days with no energy, but he forced himself to do his chores. In addition he had worsening of his chronic lung trouble and had awoken that morning feeling pins and needles sensation in his arms and legs. Chris was weaker than Amanda had ever seen him before, and she was very worried. They were willing to come to the office if I could see him right away that morning. I assured her I would see him as soon as he could come.

When Chris and Amanda arrived, I immediately noticed how thin he was. At 5' 9" tall he weighed just 135 pounds. He had no fever, and his other vital signs were normal. He told me that with the recent diarrhea he had had no fever or blood in the stool. He said that he had been weak and fatigued for two years, but it was much worse now. At thirty-two years of age Chris had had "lung trouble" almost his whole life. He had a chronic cough and was often very short of breath with audible wheezing. He had been tested for tuberculosis ten years before, but it was negative.

Surprisingly, with his long history of "lung trouble", Chris had never been diagnosed with pneumonia. It had been fifteen years since his last chest x-ray. Because of his breathing problems Chris had never been able to do woodworking or regular farming. Most of his adult life he had been a teacher in the Amish schools. He found consolation in this, as Amanda and he had never been able to have children of their own. Being childless was a real cross to bear for an Amish couple. When they moved to this area, Chris decided he would like to try raising fruits and vegetables on the small farm they had purchased. This would be his first year farming.

On examination Chris' most striking finding was the decreased breath sounds throughout his chest except for rattles and harsh sounds in the bases of both of his lungs. His abdomen showed slightly diminished bowel sounds with a mild diffuse tenderness. His legs were extremely thin, and his reflexes diminished. He was weak but able to walk. He agreed to let me get a chest x-ray on him. This showed heavy scarring in his right middle lobe, multiple granulomas like one would see in diseases such as tuberculosis, and hyperexpansion of the chest consistent with wheezing and tightness. We did a new TB skin test and drew blood for testing. I began him on an antibiotic for the diarrhea and chest findings, and I asked him to keep me informed as to how he was doing.

I didn't have to wait long. Amanda called that afternoon to report that for the past hour Chris had not been able to walk at all and now could not raise his handkerchief to his nose. I told her I would come out as soon as I finished with my present patient. She related that she remembered having read in the Budget, the Amish national newspaper, about people who had been afflicted with Guillain-Barre syndrome, and what it had done to them. She was afraid Chris might have this, too. I finished with the patient in the office, asked my nurse to cancel the rest of my afternoon and reschedule those patients, grabbed my black bag, and drove to the Yoder house.

When I arrived, Amanda met me at the door and led me to Chris, who was sitting very still in his chair. He could not raise his hand in greeting or even gesture. He said he wasn't really in pain but couldn't move much. I took the hammer out of my bag to check his reflexes once again; there was no response. Chris was indeed afflicted with Guillain-Barre syndrome and was quickly becoming paralyzed higher and higher up his body. Given how much his condition had changed in the past three hours, I knew we had no time to waste. I called the hospitalist on duty to let him know what was happening. I had Amanda prepare a small bag for him while I went to the neighbor's for help in carrying Chris out to my car. The two of us were able to load Chris into the front seat and belt him in with a pillow to help prop him up. Amanda climbed in back seat and we took off for the hospital.

Guillain-Barre syndrome is an autoimmune disorder in which the immune system makes antibodies that attack the myelin sheath, the "insulation" of the nerves. When the myelin breaks down, nerve signals cannot be transmitted, and thus paralysis ensues. Certain viruses and a few bacteria like Campylobacter can lead to this syndrome. It can even be caused by an influenza vaccination. Clearly the diarrheal illness Chris had had was the cause of his present problem. There were two ways to treat this syndrome - plasmapheresis (plasma exchange to remove the offending antibodies) or infusion of large amounts of gamma globulin. Both of these treatments appear to be equally effective.

When we arrived at the local hospital, the hospitalist then began an extensive evaluation including a spinal tap and dozens of blood tests from multiple viruses, to tick-borne illnesses, to cystic fibrosis. Three hours after admission, Chris was in ICU on a ventilator and begun on IV gamma globulin. The paralysis now involved the muscles of breathing, and he could no longer breathe on his own.

The results of the testing showed it had most likely been a coxsackie virus that started all this. Tests for lung disorders including cystic fibrosis were negative. Ultimately Chris was found to have primary ciliary dyskinesia, a hereditary disorder. Cilia are tiny hair-like structures on the cells that line our airways; they oscillate in waves to move mucus out. They are also found on certain reproductive cells. This explained Chris' lung and infertility problems. We later found out that he had two brothers similarly affected. There was no cure for this, but it could be managed once he recovered from the paralysis.

That recovery seemed long in coming. Chris was transferred to a special ventilator facility in a large city where he developed both a deep vein blood clot in his leg and pneumonia and had to be transferred to an acute care hospital for a time. It took almost two months before Chris was able to breath on his own and start to recover the control of his body. Once he could breath without the ventilator, he was sent to a nursing home near his house where he would receive continued physical and occupational therapy.

I saw Chris at the nursing home to do his admission paperwork and orders. I realized all of the care he would be getting there could be done in his own home at a substantially lower cost. He would also be back in his own home, which itself would be a big boost to his spirits. We discussed this and made arrangements for him to get the hospital bed and other equipment he would need at the house. I set up the home health services, and the next day he was discharged home. The nursing home personnel helped me load him into our van, and my wife, Dianne, and I drove him home. There several of the men from his community carried him into the house and tucked him in bed.

For the next several weeks Chris slowly continued to improve. He told me he had had several important milestones: first time to turn over in bed by himself; first time sitting up without support; first time to walk again, and so on. Chris told me one of the best was being able to go to the bathroom by himself. Perhaps the next best was being able to hold a fork or spoon and feed himself. He remarked that if any good had come from his illness, it was a deep appreciation for the ability to do all the little things he had formerly taken for granted and had suddenly lost. Chris understood how blessed he was to recover it all.

It has been almost three years since Chris' diarrhea began. He has had good and bad days with the underlying lung problems, but he is once again growing fruits and vegetables. He has his life back.

Miracle

Margaret, the Amish midwife, called Dianne and me just before 9:00 that night. She was at the house of Jacob and Katie, who had been in labor with her sixth baby for only a few hours. As the labor began to progress, Margaret had suddenly become alarmed at what she was feeling on exam. It was a protruding foot. She had been doing this work for several decades and had delivered more babies than most doctors, so I knew I could trust her judgment. I advised her we'd come out right away.

What Margaret had described over the phone is known as a footling breech. These babies are in a breech position, bottom down, and one leg is extended so that the foot can be clearly felt as the presenting part of the baby. As a result, there is a high incidence of "cord accidents". The umbilical cord drops down along the leg and gets pinched, cuts off the baby's oxygen, and the baby dies. These babies cannot be delivered safely in the normal way. Cesarean section is required. Fortunately the footling breech presentation is relatively rare. My wife, Dianne, a registered nurse, had worked in labor and delivery for almost thirty years and saw very few of these cases. This was only the second footling breech I had seen in over twenty-five years of delivering babies. Maybe I had just been lucky.

Dianne and I drove to the house of Jacob and Katie. It was pitch dark with no moon. As soon as we went inside, Margaret led us to the bedroom where Katie was laboring. A quick examination confirmed what she had found. This baby was a footling breech. There was no possibility of a safe home delivery. Although all five of their other children had been born at home with no problems or complications, this time was different. I discussed what was happening with both Katie and Jacob. They understood the life-threatening risk to the baby and agreed that Katie would be taken to the hospital for a Cesarean delivery. Before they would go to the hospital, though, they wanted to talk with her father, the bishop. I understood she meant he would come to pray over them and the baby.

While the bishop was being notified, I called the OB floor and spoke with one of the obstetricians in town, who happened to be there with another delivery. I explained to him that Katie's case was a footling breech. He advised me to get her to the hospital right away and not wait for her father to come. I decided we would honor Jacob and Katie's wishes instead and wait for the bishop. Prayer can have a powerful influence in our lives, and all of us felt this baby could use all the help he could get. I think those prayers were crucial.

When the bishop arrived, he already had been told what was happening. He led the family in prayers. When he was finished, we all helped Katie into our van and drove to the hospital with her, Jacob, Margaret, and the bishop. It was one of those times we were glad we had Dianne's van and not my PT Cruiser! We drove up to the emergency entrance, and I got Katie a wheelchair. We wheeled her into the hospital, and when the ER personnel saw we had a lady in labor, they directed us to go directly to OB while Jacob stayed to register her.

Arriving at the labor unit we handed Katie over to the nurses working there while I again briefed the obstetrician on what I had discovered at the house. Once Katie was in bed, he went into her room and checked her again. He came out of the room looking doubtfully at Margaret and me. He said he found the baby was breech but did not feel a foot. Margaret and I looked at each other for a moment in disbelief. Each of us knew we had felt a baby's foot. He felt that the baby might be able to have a breech delivery without a C- section and wanted to watch her for a while. We assured him we had both felt the foot, but he insisted it was not there now. He asked me to check her again and see if I felt a foot. He was right; the foot I had felt before was not there! I explained to him that her exam had changed. He told us that he had never seen a footling breech withdraw the foot back up into the uterus. Again we advised him that both of us had felt the foot and had no doubts that this had been a footling breech. He thought about it a moment, then decided to go ahead with the C-section.

By then Jacob was at his wife's bedside. The obstetrician explained to them that what he had found on exam was not what Margaret and I had found earlier. Nevertheless, trusting our judgment, and given that the baby was still breech, he recommended a C-section. He explained the procedure and the reasons for it. Katie sign the consent form. Meanwhile, the nurses were on the telephone calling in the C-section crew and getting the operating room set up; there was little time to waste in getting everything ready.

The obstetrician asked me to assist with the surgery. We both changed into surgical scrubs and began scrubbing for the procedure while the anesthetist was giving Katie an epidural anaesthetic. We came into the room, gowned and gloved, and draped Katie for the surgery. When all was ready, the C-section began in the usual way - open the skin, then the uterus, then deliver the baby.

However, this time just as the obstetrician was preparing to deliver the baby, the baby's placenta spontaneously sheared off the wall of the uterus. This is a life-threatening condition called abruption, the treatment for which is immediate emergency C-section. Had this occurred at home, we would have lost both the baby and Katie. It was a miracle the abruption did not happen until the very moment the obstetrician was already delivering the baby!

The bishop's prayers had had a powerful effect!

Amish Wedding

We missed the wedding. The bishop, Eli, went to a neighbor and called when the ceremony was finished, as that was the soonest he could contact us. He had just presided at the wedding of his daughter Lydia and Aaron, the young man who had been courting her. Eli told us that van loads of people from both families had come from out of state for this wedding, and among them was a sick baby. He asked us to come and see this child. Dianne and I promised to be there shortly.

Amish weddings are usually held on Thursdays in the fall. They are serious but very joyful affairs, the actual service taking about three hours. Practically all of it is prescribed, so the bride is not harried with planning her wedding like "English" brides do. This tradition gives the young couple more time to ponder the serious step they are taking. Marriage is a lifelong commitment; divorce is almost unheard of among the Amish. After the long service, everyone converges on the home of the bride where the newlyweds are seated in a specially prepared corner of the front room, and the feast begins. It is considered a special honor to sit beside the new couple ("side sitters"), be a waiter, a cook or a hostler ("park" everyone's horses). Often those who serve in such capacities are mentioned in the Budget newspaper. Each community has a scribe who receives the paper free in exchange for submitting the news.

The bishop's long lane was crowded. There were twenty vans parked all around the house and down the lane. We had to park out by the main road and walk the two-hundred yards up to the house. Dianne carried my black bag while I carried the heavier soft luggage in which I kept the medications for dispensing. I was glad it was a pleasantly cool autumn day.

As we approached the first barn, we saw a dozen or so youths in their early teens standing talking by the van in which they had come. As we passed, one of the older boys, speaking in the Swiss dialect, made a disparaging remark to his friends about the "English" and doctors. For a moment they chuckled softly amongst themselves, until I said in the Swiss dialect, "Gip acht! E ken de Doddy." (Watch out! I know your father.) The speaker's eyes grew wide and a look of fear passed over his face. He had had no idea that I could understand exactly what he had said!

As we continued on past the first barn, we came to an open grassy area between the barns where large numbers of young adults were trying to play a volleyball game. I use the word "trying" since there must have been twenty or more people on each side of the net. It didn't matter, though, as they were all laughing and having a great time. In about another ten paces we had come to the back of the food line. We were still more than twenty yards from the house.

As we walked past those waiting to eat, I began wondering how we were going to find the sick baby we were supposed to see. Dianne asked me how we would find this baby in so large a crowd. I suggested we go the rest of the way up to the house and look for the bishop. Before we could get close to the door, a young couple walked up to us holding their sick child. They had been in a group on the other side of the house, yet word we'd arrived was passed up the line, through the house, and out to them faster than we could even walk up to the house!

The baby was eight months old and had had a cold for six days. Now he was running a fever. We walked over where the church benches had been set up in the shade by the house. Setting down the medication bag, I pulled out a blank chart and the thermometer. While I began making notes on the baby, Dianne took his temperature. He had a fever of 101.8° under the arm. I looked into my black bag for the diagnostic tools to check his ears and throat. When I looked up, I found we had been suddenly surrounded by dozens of small children eager to watch what we were doing. I had never had such an audience watch me examine a patient!

The baby's eyes were slightly reddened, and his nose was congested with thick yellow-green mucus. Examination showed what Dianne and I had both suspected, middle ear infections in both ears. I asked for a glass of water to prepare a liquid antibiotic for the baby. His parents then paid me for the visit and the medicine, and we began to pack up our supplies to leave. Before we could even get things back in the bags, another couple approached us asking if I was the doctor the bishop had called. When I said I was, they asked us to stay to see their five year-old daughter, too. She had been sick and started running a fever just that day. We agreed.

The second couple's daughter proved to have tonsillitis. Once again I mixed up an appropriate antibiotic. Her parents were still writing the check for the call and the medication when the next couple walked up with a sick child. We ended up seeing six sick children, one after another, only one of which lived in the local community. When we had finished seeing all six, we finally packed up everything and were about to leave when Eli walked up to thank us for having come so quickly. He then insisted we share in the wedding meal before going home. It was a bit embarrassing when he led us to the front of the line, but we had no choice.

It was a wonderful meal with more kinds of good food than we could possibly sample, but everyone urged us to try it all. After eating we congratulated the newlyweds before finally walking back to the car for the drive back to town. As we walked down the lane to the car, we passed again the young man who had made the earlier remark about doctors. I turned to him and said, "De Doddy het tsate, 'Settlsh abba!'" (Your father said, "You settle down!")

The look on his face was almost as satisfying as the wedding meal itself.

Pre-Eclampsia

Margaret, the midwife, called me about her granddaughter, Anna, who was expecting her second child. Anna's father was the bishop. Margaret told me she had a "little high blood pressure" and a "little protein" in her urine. She told me Anna was due in about a week, and Margaret wondered if I could come out to see her. That afternoon I drove out to the bishop's farm to see the patient.

When I arrived, I was greeted by the dog, actually named Rover, and the bishop himself. He and his wife knew that their daughter was developing a serious problem and were glad I had come. Anna was a very quiet but self-assured young lady who did not seem upset about her condition. I could not tell if she was unaware of the risks to her and the baby, or if she was simply taking them in stride.

We began by collecting a urine specimen to test again. This time her urine showed no evidence for infection, but there was significant protein present. I measured her blood pressure and found it was 162/112, which was much too high. She told me she had started on her own taking the left-over blood pressure medicine prescribed during her first pregnancy. That child was two years old, so the medicine was even older. It had lost its potency and was not working for her as it had with the previous pregnancy. I checked her reflexes, and they were normal. Her legs were not swollen with fluid. Her baby was active with a normal pulse and in good position for delivery.

Anna was experiencing pre-eclampsia, a complication of pregnancy characterized by high blood pressure, progressively increasing protein in the urine, fluid retention, and brisk reflexes. Untreated, it can lead to eclampsia, in which the mother has generalized seizures. Eclampsia can cause the death of both mother and baby. Anna was clearly in moderate to severe pre-eclampsia and needed treatment. Ideally she would be hospitalized, given magnesium intravenously, and delivered with induction of labor if needed.

Surrounded by the bishop, his wife, Anna and her husband, his parents, and the midwife, I began to explain to them how serious her condition was. Proper treatment meant hospitalizing Anna that day and beginning the indicated treatment. Anna would not agree, and her husband and all the grandparents supported this decision. As the bishop put it, "That's not our way." I would learn over the coming years how concerned they were about costs, willing to accept even death rather than run up a large debt. After all, this life was just a stepping stone to the next and needn't be preserved at all costs.

Now I felt I was in a real bind ethically. I would be held to a standard of care which my patient would not accept. I had made clear the risks to Anna and her baby, and everyone expressed understanding. Yet Anna was adamant that she would not go to the hospital. She insisted she did not feel bad and that she would just get more rest at home. She agreed to let me prescribe the blood pressure medication again, and she promised to take it. But she flatly refused hospital care. Margaret assured me that she would check Anna's blood pressure every day and make sure she was resting. When I asked her directly if she agreed that she should be hospitalized, she just shrugged her shoulders without saying anything.

Unable to convince Anna to accept the standard of care, I had no alternative but to have her sign a statement stating the risks she was taking and that she was insisting on doing so. In addition to this I felt I had enough witnesses in the group that I had done my best to try to convince her. I called the prescription for her medication to a pharmacy in town and left with the promise to return in a week to recheck her. As I drove home, I could not stop worrying whether I had done the right thing. I knew some of my colleagues would have simply washed their hands of her as a patient when Anna would not cooperate with standard care. Yet I felt I couldn't abandon her as a patient. Concern for the patient exceeded concern for the consequences of her decision. By not putting her in the hospital I felt I was leaving us both in jeopardy with Anna, of course, taking the greater risk.

Each day for the next week I waited in anticipation for the phone call from Margaret relating Anna's blood pressure and overall condition. Her blood pressure came down somewhat during the week after she had begun the blood pressure medication, but she continued to have protein in the urine. By Thursday she began showing swelling in her ankles; this was much worse the following day. That Friday evening I went out to check her again.

Once more I found myself facing the same crowd with whom I had talked a week before. Again I went over the signs of pre-eclampsia and again stressed the need to initiate treatment and induce labor. Her blood pressure was a little lower, but the presence of the swelling was worrisome. Her pre-eclampsia was worse. Still Anna would not accept the standard of care for this problem. I must have gone over everything at least twice, and I could see her parents and husband weren't so sure this time. They began to talk with Anna in the German, which I had not yet learned. It was a strange feeling to be explaining things as a physician, then suddenly become an outsider to the conversation.

After a few minutes they all turned back to me. Anna said she would agree to go to the hospital on Monday if she did not deliver before then. I told her that my wife, Dianne, an OB nurse for many years, had told me many times that there were always more deliveries during bad thunderstorms, though this might just be nurses' superstition. I told Anna that while I was driving to their house, I had heard on the radio that the forecast for the weekend was for rain. Maybe she would have this baby at home after all. If not, I would arrange for her admission Monday morning.

Saturday dawned a cool clear day, but by late morning the sky became cloudy. That afternoon we had a fierce thunderstorm. The rain was heavy for several hours with frequent crashing lightning. I hoped that Dianne's remark about storms and labor was right. I still had my doubts that I was doing the right thing, yet I knew I had no right to "commit" health care on Anna when she would not accept the standard treatment.

Sunday morning the phone rang. It was Anna's husband. He told me Anna had delivered during the night. Now her blood pressure was down almost to normal, and the swelling was going down, too.

I wasn't sure who to thank first - God, the weatherman, or my wife. What I had been told by the last two had been right: we did have a thunderstorm, and the thunderstorm "superstition" had worked. Both Anna and I could finally rest easy.

Rib Click

Josiah Hochstetler was just three weeks old. He had been delivered by a midwife at home, and his mother, Catherine, said there were no problems or special difficulties with the delivery. He was nursing well and gaining weight, but he had a peculiar problem. At times he would have an audible "pop" in his chest. She had first noticed this when he was just a few hours old and nursing. She had never had anything like this with any of her other six children. She and her husband, Eli, had decided to wait a little while to see if it would go away. She was calling me as it had not.

Eli and Catherine had just recently moved into the community from Ohio. It was a difficult time for Catherine, as she was close to term, but they made the trip here with all their household goods without problems. With help from the people in the new settlement they had unpacked and settled in. A former neighbor of theirs from Ohio had moved here earlier, and knowing someone already here had eased the transition for them and the children. Josiah had been born in their new home just a month after the move.

I drove out to the Hochstetler home to see Josiah. Catherine came to the door holding him. We went into the main room where she laid him down for me to examine. He was apparently in no distress now, though Catherine said that initially the popping sound did seem to bother him. As I began to examine him, I was wondering if this "pop" might happen while I was there. I need not have worried; within moments I heard and felt this peculiar pop.

The sound and a clicking sensation were coming from the junction of one of his right lower ribs with the sternum, or breastbone. This was an area that would not become calcified or show up on an x-ray for many months to come. The skin overlying this area was completely normal, and there were no bruises anywhere on his skin. His lungs were clear on examination, and except for the strange popping, his examination was entirely normal. He even had almost no jaundice, unusual for a breast-fed baby this young.

In my training we had been taught how to check the newborn for a hip click, a sound coming from a congenitally loose hip joint. The babies so affected would have their legs braced with splints or a cast to hold the hips in position while the joint finished developing. Once the hip was held tightly in place, the splinting could be stopped. Yet I had never heard of a "rib click" before. I assured Catherine that this was not dangerous and should resolve on its own. I told her I would try to get some printed information about this condition and send it to her.

As I drove back to town, I kept wondering whether there was any information available on this condition. Certainly I could not recall ever having seen this before, but I did seem to recall having heard of it. In thinking about sources for information about this, I decided to try the internet and search for general articles about this. Surely that would give me what I was looking for.

When I got back to town, I stopped at the hospital to look up "rib click" on the internet. Much to my consternation, I was unable to find any information about such a phenomenon in newborns. There were several articles about similar rib problems in adults but nothing regarding newborns. I tried many other search terms trying to get information I could share with Josiah's parents, but I was unable to locate any information on this topic by using the internet.

Just in case I might have missed something during my training, I left the hospital and returned to the office to search my old pediatric textbooks. Surely the section on examination of the normal newborn would discuss this finding, but no, nothing was written about clicking ribs, just hips. Finally I thought I had better call the local pediatrician to see what he knew about this.

The pediatrician told me he had never heard of such a finding. He was suspicious that the baby might have been injured or abused. He suggested I get an immediate bone survey, x-rays of all the baby's bones, looking for fractures or other signs of child abuse. To be fair, this pediatrician had spent many years working in a major city hospital where child abuse was unfortunately far too common. As a result, I felt his outlook might be a bit skewed. Having worked with Amish patients for many years and observing the Hochstetler family in particular, I could not accept abuse as a cause for this unusual finding.

Finally, I called the big children's hospital to which our hospital referred newborns with problems. I explained to the resident on call what I had found and asked if she knew about this or had seen it before. She said she had never heard of it but would ask their two neonatogists, specialists in newborn care, what they thought. They had never seen a case like this either. They said if child abuse was not an issue, the baby still needed the bone survey looking for other fractures. They reminded me of something I had seen before, though only once - osteogenesis imperfecta.

Osteogenesis imperfecta is a genetic disorder in which the bones do not calcify normally. They are very thin and can be fractured with just a slight bump. This disorder is detected in the first months of life when the baby can't be comforted, and the parents don't know why. X-rays show very thin bones and often multiple fractures in various stages of healing. This condition can sometimes be confused with child abuse, but there is one glaring difference. In child abuse the bones are calcified normally, but in osteogenesis imperfecta they are not. Also, in this condition the whites of the eyes are very often a deep robin's egg blue.

Once again I drove to the Hochstetler home, this time to get Josiah x-rayed. His parents understood my concern, and Catherine remembered knowing of a girl where she had lived before who was affected with the genetic disease. They agreed to the x-rays. I drove Catherine and Josiah to the hospital for the bone survey while Eli stayed at home with the other children. As soon as the x-rays were completed, I introduced Catherine to the radiologist and had him check Josiah's rib. He was just as surprised as I had been when the rib clicked for him. The x-rays showed little Josiah had normally calcified bones and no fractures. Clearly he had neither been abused nor afflicted with osteogenesis imperfecta. He just had a rib click. I mentioned to Catherine on the way back to their house that we were bothered by the rib click a lot more than he was!

It was a month later that I attended a lecture by a visiting expert on child abuse. Afterward I asked the speaker if she had ever heard of a rib click. Indeed, she replied, she had heard of a case like this once before. The child was just as untroubled by it as Josiah was and outgrew it in the first year of life. That child was at first misdiagnosed as abused. Having learned this, I was able to reassure the Hochstetlers that Josiah would be fine. He just clicked!

Made in the USA
Lexington, KY
28 April 2013